Janet Balaskas is the mother of three classes for mothers and fathers-to-be London. She was trained by the Natio childbirth educator and has since pioneered a new approach to pre-natal preparation and birth.

She launched a national campaign to establish parents' rights to choose a natural active birth. In 1982 she organized the highly successful 'Birthrights Rally' and two International Conferences on Active Birth. She is the founder of the Active Birth Movement.

Janet is the co-author of *New Life*, written together with her husband Arthur in 1979, and has since written *Active Birth* and made a video film also entitled *Active Birth* as well as a radio/cassette called *Shape up for Motherhood*.

Other books by Janet Balaskas

New Life (with Arthur Balaskas)
Active Birth

Author's Acknowledgements

I would like to thank Sarah and Francis Payne and Gigi and Alan White for so generously donating the photographs and also all the men and women with whom I have shared the experiences that make up this book. Thanks also to all the members of the Active Birth Movement for their pioneering work, help and support over the years.

The Active Birth Partners Handbook

JANET BALASKAS

Foreword by Yehudi Gordon
Introduction by Arthur Balaskas

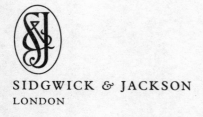

SIDGWICK & JACKSON
LONDON

First published in Great Britain by
Sidgwick & Jackson Limited

This revised edition published in October 1986
First reprint October 1987
Second reprint August 1989

The author and publishers are grateful for
permission to reproduce the line illustrations on
pages 22, 23 (top and bottom right), 24 (right), 26,
29, 32, 82, 83, 97 and 98, which are by Laura
McKechnie and originally appeared in *Active Birth*
by Janet Balaskas, published by Unwin Paperbacks in 1983.
Those on pages 19 and 21 are by Janet
Balaskas and originally appeared in *New Life*,
published by Sidgwick & Jackson in 1979. All the
other line drawings are by Claudio Munoz

The black and white photographs were taken by
Anthea Sieveking (Vision International)

Design by Lynda Smith

ISBN 0-283-99441-X

Typeset by Tellgate Limited, London WC2
Printed and bound in Great Britain by
Biddles Limited, Guildford and King's Lynn
for Sidgwick & Jackson Limited
1 Tavistock Chambers, Bloomsbury Way
London WC1A 2SG

Author's Preface to the Second Edition

A modern woman giving birth today does so in a social context which has no historical precedent. In times gone by the birth of a child usually took place within the family, and the mother would probably have been attended by a midwife, and close women friends or female relatives. In such a context the secrets and skills of motherhood and birth were passed on down the generations as a natural heritage.

In this century rapid social change has had a powerful effect on the way we live and the way we are born. Birth has become primarily a medical event, usually taking place within the unfamiliar environment of a hospital, subject to the current trends and latest advances in obstetric health care. Changes in lifestyle have left most women separated by a 'generation gap' from their own mothers and living at a distance from their friends and relatives.

The person to whom the pregnant women is closest is usually the man with whom she is living, and it is not surprising that it has become both customary and necessary for many modern women to be accompanied by their partner when giving birth. Sometimes that partner may be someone other than the father of the baby, such as a close friend or relative or a birth counsellor with whom she chooses to share the experience.

The prospect of being present at a birth can be awesome, particularly if all you have to go on is a secondary school biology course. For this reason a new custom of preparing for the birth of a child by attending a course of classes during pregnancy has evolved over the past few decades. At first these were designed for women only, and fathers were invited for perhaps one evening at the end of the course. Now, with the growing recognition of the importance of the partner's role in the birth, these courses have expanded to include participation by partners, so that anyone intending to be present at a birth can begin this sharing during the pregnancy. This affords him or her the opportunity to approach the experience with understanding and

insight and also to learn how to be helpful in an effective, yet unob-
trusive way. This is especially important to the father who wishes to
take an active role in the birth of his child and to share in the intimacy
and privacy of the experience with the mother. To her the father's
presence may be vitally necessary as the one person on whom she can
depend and who will be able to understand her needs in labour.

Over the years I have greatly enjoyed providing such courses for
pregnant women and their partners. It is a special pleasure to observe
the men in these groups making the challenging transition into
fatherhood. Years later many of them have told me that being there
to welcome their baby from the start was a deeply meaningful and
moving experience which created a lasting closeness to their newborn child. After the birth I am often told how invaluable the father's
presence and support was to the mother, and how helpful it was to
begin the adventure of parenthood by preparing together for the
birth.

This preparation is especially relevant to women who would like
to have an active natural birth, and will need the help and support of
their partners in order to feel relaxed, secure and free enough to
achieve this in an environment which may not always be ideal.

This book is a condensed version of the topics we usually cover in
a partner's course and is written especially from the partner's point of
view. Although a book could never replace the course itself, I hope
that the practical information and encouragement it contains will be
an enjoyable and helpful guide to starting a family.

Janet Balaskas
August 1986

Contents

Foreword by Yehudi Gordon

I am very pleased to write the Foreword for Janet Balaskas's book on the role of the partner in Active Birth. It is a welcome addition to the bibliography on birth because there is a distinct need at the present time for this volume. Having a baby is an important event in the life cycle and today's parents, who are better informed than ever before and who increasingly recognize the importance of a good start in life, expect and deserve a choice and the right to celebrate the birth of their children in a way which is safe and satisfying.

Many men want to be intimately involved at all stages of planning for the pregnancy, in supporting their women through the gestation period and during the labour and birth and in caring for their children. Men often feel ineffectual in the domain of pregnancy and birth and, while wanting to be helpful and involved, may feel frustrated and even neglected.

A number of books have been written but this book is exceptional in, amongst other things, providing massage and yoga-based exercises for couples to practise together, thus using touch and stretching as an additional means of communication. Women who have not done any exercise for years suddenly find that the ante-natal yoga exercises are making them fitter than they have ever been prior to their pregnancy.

The advantages of this type of preparation are numerous: natural, upright positions for birth make maximum use of gravity and allow the weight of the baby to increase the expulsive force during birth; the upright posture reduces the degree of pain and distress for the mother, making the time between contractions longer and the force of each contraction more positive. The mother's hormonal secretions are undisturbed and her uterus can work without unnecessary resistance resulting in a decreased need for pain relief. Equally important are the psychological advantages for the mother, father and newborn baby. The preparation advocated in this book for the birth and care of a child is likely to make the event more relaxed and more loving.

This book is in keeping with Janet Balaskas's philosophy that people should be encouraged, in a warm, friendly and sympathetic way, to care for themselves and to take responsibility for the birth and development of their children. Active Birth is not new and has been practised throughout the world for millenia. Parents, midwives and obstetricians have always been aware of the importance of emotional and physical health to encourage normal development of the baby and to assist the birth. The use of yoga–based stretching exercises and massage often puts people in touch with their bodies and builds their confidence and makes a happy outcome more likely.

As a Consultant Obstetrician and father of three children, I feel that men who read this book and experiment with the exercises will have gained a number of things. They will understand the changes their women experience during pregnancy and birth, they will feel more confident about helping their women to prepare for the birth and about assisting during the birth itself. They will also feel good about touching and stretching their babies after birth. Therefore, this book is a must for all fathers who wish to participate in Active Birth and parenting.

Yehudi Gordon
January 1984

Introduction by Arthur Balaskas

Why is such a book as this one necessary? The answer is simply to end the state of ignorance about childbirth which most men are in.

Fifteen years ago, I was under the impression that when his woman was with child, a man's only responsibility was to find the best professional in the field. My family's advice was never to stint when you needed a lawyer, accountant or doctor. My first wife and I were in London and so to a Harley Street specialist she went. She experienced the full, modern obstetric treatment – that is: induction, lying on her back, anaesthetic, forceps, episiotomy and so on. I was told that I was the father of a baby girl and called in to see her and my wife.

My first look at our baby daughter stopped my breath. She had black marks all around her face and head. The nurse noticed my shock and quickly put me straight.

'Don't be so alarmed,' she said, 'they aren't birth marks, only bruises from the forceps.'

A little later I questioned the obstetrician about how the birth went. 'No complication, quite routine,' he said.

Right there and then I somehow instinctively felt, first of all, that there must be other more natural ways to bring a child into this world. I realized that my wife had not 'given birth' but had gone through some kind of 'extraction'. Secondly, I thought, surely a father could participate in this crucial event if he wanted to?

This book, written by Janet, stems from our personal experiences and focuses on these points. It encourages a woman to actively 'give birth' in the full sense, and it guides and prepares a man to participate. *The Active Birth Partners Handbook* is for men who want to take part responsibly in the birth of their children. It is the kind of fathers' book that every expectant mother, midwife or birth attendant will also want to read. It is an intelligently written, challenging guide for anyone helping a woman give birth in a natural, intuitive, sensible way.

13

The opening chapter builds a strong and true case for encouraging women to have complete freedom in selecting bodily positions during labour and childbirth, and it suggests feeling the bony passages through which the child will be born in order to understand the physiology of an active birth. The next chapter discusses pregnancy – from conception, through the baby's development in the womb, to the time immediately prior to birth. Chapter 3 is on stretching exercises, the simplest and most effective way of relaxing the body. As Janet quite rightly says, you and your partner have a great chance during the months of pregnancy not only to prepare for the birth but also to benefit yourselves through the practice of stretching and breathing exercises. All her suggestions are simple and effective. Next comes a chapter on massage, where it is suggested that before beginning to massage your partner you should work on your own body. The chapter on labour and birth is the focal point for her advice, and this guide to labour and delivery is very useful indeed. Knowing beforehand the possibilities involved in the hours of birthing and the final birth is a must. Chapter 6 outlines the environment for birth and lays out the choices with all their pros and cons. Then there is a chapter on the unexpected so that if there are any complications you are not suddenly left in the dark. The book ends with a chapter on what happens after the birth – from the first minutes and hours, through the first days, ending with ways to handle and play with your child later on.

Janet knows her subject. She has herself given birth actively to our two children and over the years has prepared hundreds of women and men to do the same. As a partner you could not do better than to practise and follow the simple and direct common sense of *The Active Birth Partners Handbook*.

Skiloundia, Greece
March 1984

1 Why an active birth?

Expressed in the simplest terms an active birth means that the woman in labour has the freedom to use her body as she chooses. She may wish to walk, stand up, kneel or squat during her contractions and when she gives birth to her baby. In fact she is most unlikely to want to lie down on her back. Lying down or semi-reclining she is helpless, like a stranded beetle, and unable to use her body to assist the descent of her baby or to make herself more comfortable. She is also in a position of surrender to obstetric intervention and far more likely to need it!

Birth in perspective

If one studies the history of childbirth one soon discovers that active birth is nothing new. Women all over the world have used a variety of upright postures to labour and give birth since prehistoric times. Similarly, amongst primitive cultures today women stand, walk, kneel or squat during labour and birth.

Modern obstetrics has its roots in seventeenth-century France, dating from around the time when forceps were invented. With the use of forceps physicians obviously preferred women to lie down for birth and in the latter part of the century it became the most popular choice for ladies of fashion, difficult as this is to believe in an age which did not possess our modern methods of pain relief! The birthstool (a chair with a horseshoe shaped seat for the mother to sit upright to give birth), at one time an essential part of a midwife's equipment, had disappeared totally by the eighteenth century. The time-honoured profession and art of midwifery declined as male physicians took over as the primary attendants of women in labour.

In the late nineteenth century chloroform was introduced as a general anaesthetic for childbirth, Queen Victoria being one of the first to try it. So in a mere two hundred years, following a heritage of active birth which had lasted for thousands, women were not only flat on their backs but unconscious too!

The twentieth century has seen two revolutions in childbirth. The first relates to modern obstetrics which has developed to such a degree that it is now possible to induce and control birth with synthetic hormones and to eradicate all sensation completely with modern methods of analgesia. We are also better ensured than ever against death in childbirth. Today, throughout the Western world, the active management of labour is used routinely. Birth has become a medical event and most couples choose to have their babies born in hospital.

The second revolution stems directly from the first. Many parents and their attendants have been dissatisfied with this obstetric take-over. Given that over 90 per cent of all births, if well managed, are potentially uncomplicated, the statistics shown by modern obstetric hospitals are very disappointing. (See the table 'Some Comparative Statistics' on page 17.) It seems that the more sophisticated the routinely applied obstetric technology, the greater the need for intervention, reaching the extreme shown in some countries, like the USA and Canada, where the Caesarean rate is almost 40 per cent in many places.

As this century has progressed, women and their partners have united in small groups throughout the world to oppose the enforced use of obstetric intervention. They have been supported by some members of the attendant professions and a new profession, that of the ante-natal teacher or birth counsellor, has developed. Fathers have demanded the right to be present and to participate in not only the birth but also the care of their children.

Today this revolution is developing apace as more couples are insisting on the right to have their babies naturally. As the attendant risks of the drugs used in labour have become better known many women have attempted to do without them. To help themselves achieve a natural birth without medication women began to use

SOME COMPARATIVE STATISTICS

The following statistics were quoted by Marsden G. Wagner of the World Health Organization at the Active Birth Conference in 1982 from his paper 'The Obstetrical Drama':

Forceps deliveries in England, Scotland and Wales	13·3%
Operative intervention in England and Wales (meaning forceps, vacuum extraction or Caearean section)	20·6%
Operative intervention in Scotland	23·7%
Induction of labour in Britain	20–30%
Episiotomy in Britain	30–90%

Statistics of the number of babies needing special care after birth in Great Britain, taken from *Perinatal Morbidity and Mortailty in Private Obstetric Practice* **by Martin Richards:**

At home	1·3%
NHS consultant bed	16·6%
NHS GP unit	7·9%
GP maternity unit	2·3%
Private	8·9%

Statistics from Michel Odent's hospital in Pithiviers, France, where all women are encouraged to give birth actively. The total number of births from January 1982 to June 1983 was 1,402:

	number of births	percentage of the total
Caesarean sections	93	6·6%
Vacuum extractions	73	5·2%
Episiotomies	84	6%
Forceps	0	0
Babies needing special care	22	1·5%

relaxation and breathing methods and to rely on the support and help of their partners. They were still, however, taking to bed during labour and using the reclining or semi-reclining position for delivery.

In the last few decades, however, in a few places in England, France, the USA, Australia, and South America women have been encouraged to use upright postures and to give birth actively, while researchers have observed the difference. As the table on page 17 shows, their statistics have revealed a significant improvement when birth is natural and, better still, active, so proving conclusively that an active birth is not only more comfortable and enjoyable for the mother but also safer for her and her baby. In Holland, where intervention is far less common than in other countries and the majority of women give birth at home, the statistics are among the best in the Western world.

So we can conclude that for scientific and medical reasons alone there is a strong case for active birth.

Another very important consideration is that of the quality of the experience of birth for the mother, father, baby and the family into which the child is born. Developments in the field of psychiatry and psychology this century have highlighted the importance of the birth experience in the life cycle of a human being. A newborn baby is exquisitely sensitive at the time of birth and can be deeply disturbed for life by any unnecessary trauma. Studies have also shown that the uninterrupted bonding between mother, newborn baby and other members of the family immediately after the birth can be a great help in the foundation of their future relationships.

Sometimes, if a medical complication arises or the baby is distressed, the natural continuity and physiology of birth has to be disturbed by intervention or the use of drugs. No one will deny that our first aim is a live, healthy mother and baby, but all too often the problems that arise in labour are caused by the intervention itself. (For example the rate of forceps deliveries amongst women who have epidurals is 20 per cent higher.) Giving birth actively reduces the need for such intervention and therefore increases the possibility of an uncomplicated birth. With mother and baby undrugged, alert and physically active circumstances are at their best.

Birth is a momentous experience for everyone and it should be a deep and joyous celebration of new life within the family. It is, after all, the fruit of love and the climactic part of a couple's sexual life.

When birth is managed routinely by obstetric intervention in a busy hospital setting, quite often this aspect is completely forgotten or actually obliterated. We do not know but can only wonder how deeply this affects our society.

Birth is primarily a natural biological function for which a woman's body is ideally designed. Although problems or disasters do occasionally occur – and we must at all times be ready for this possibility – the vast majority of births are potentially without complication. Every woman, like any other animal, has the instinctive knowledge of how to give birth within her own body. By literally confining her to the recumbent or semi-reclining position we are denying her the power to use these instincts. Unless she is lucky enough to have a very easy birth, she will be completely dependant on the help and intervention of others to deliver her baby.

The physiology of an active birth

THE PELVIS

In order to understand the basic physiology let us study the pelvis, or bony passage through which the baby has to pass as he is born.

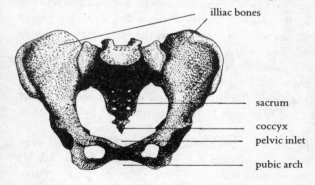

illiac bones

sacrum

coccyx
pelvic inlet

pubic arch

The female pelvis

Try this

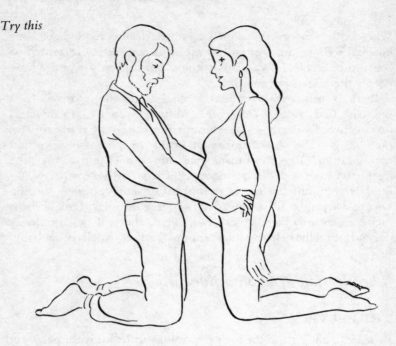

Working with your partner place your hands on her hips and find the corners or iliac bones of the two hips at her sides. Pressing gently with your thumbs, explore the top rim of the hip bones until you come to the centre of her lower back where they join the spine.

Next place your palm, fingers down, over the base of her spine and feel the sacrum which forms the back wall of the pelvis. Pressing with your fingertips, feel the coccyx or tailbone at the base of the spine. Then use your fingertips to feel the top of the pubic bone in front.

As it begins its journey through the birth canal, the baby's head will fit snugly in the round pelvic inlet at the top. As the labour progresses the head will descend deeper into the pelvic canal, gradually rotating as it moves down. By the time it reaches the floor of the pelvis it will have turned, ready to be born, through the pelvic outlet at the base of the pelvis.

Basically the pelvis is a curved funnel.

The pelvic canal

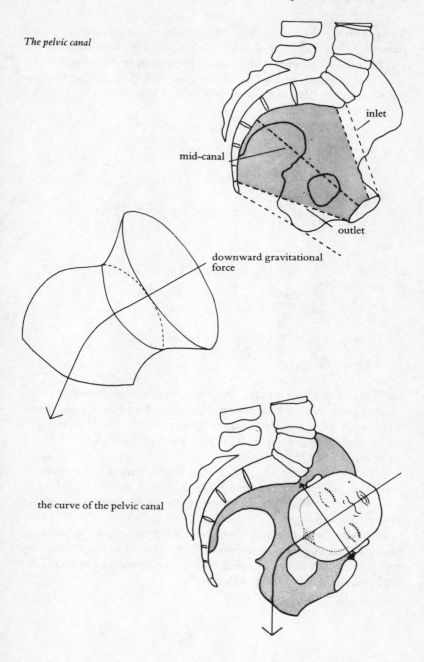

inlet

mid–canal

outlet

downward gravitational force

the curve of the pelvic canal

Just as you would hold a funnel up to pour water through it, so the passage of the baby through the pelvis will be much easier if the mother is in an upright position when the downward force of gravity can assist the child's progress. If the mother is lying on her back or semi-reclining this has the same effect as if you tried to pour water sideways through a funnel.

The pelvic joints

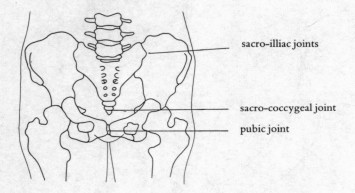

sacro–illiac joints

sacro–coccygeal joint

pubic joint

The pelvis has four joints. During pregnancy a woman's body secretes hormones which soften these in order to make the pelvis more expandable and elastic for the birth.

The *pubic joint* in front can open as much as ½ inch in labour to make more space for the baby.

The *sacro-coccygial joint* lies between the tailbone and the sacrum. This is normally fused but for birth it softens so that the tailbone can rotate out of the way as the baby's head comes through. A very good reason not to sit on it!

The two *sacro-iliac joints* lie between the hip bones and the sacrum. They expand sideways to some extent to widen the canal but more importantly they have a pivot-like action which has a significant part to play in the descent of the baby.

The pivotal axis of the sacro-illiac joint

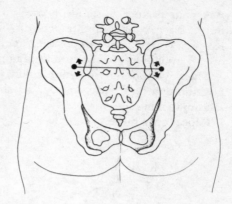

Try this

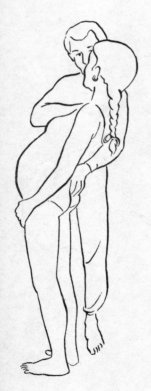

Leaning back the pelvic outlet closes

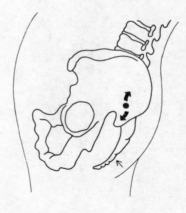

Ask your partner to stand or kneel in an upright position on the floor. Place your palm, fingers down, firmly over her sacrum. Keeping your hand in this position, ask her to bend forward from the hips. You will feel her sacrum lifting up.

Then, without moving your hand, ask her to return to an upright position and lean back slightly. As she does so you will feel her sacrum tucking in.

Repeat once more.

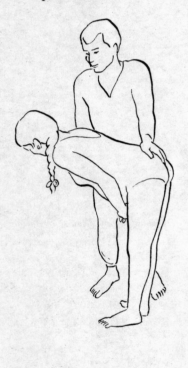

Leaning forward the pelvic outlet opens

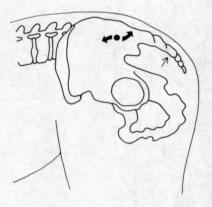

When your partner leans forward her sacrum lifts and opens the pelvic outlet: when she leans back it tucks in and the size of the outlet is considerably reduced. Now ask her to adopt the semi-reclining position. Place your hands under her lower back and you will feel that her entire weight is resting on her sacrum in this position, closing it to its maximum. In terms of opening she could hardly be in a more disadvantageous position!

During labour and birth if the mother stands, kneels or squats, her trunk leans forward and the birth canal opens. If she lies back it closes. In fact, studies which have compared the semi-reclining position to squatting (in which the pelvis is at its most open) show that there can be a loss of up to 30 per cent of the possible opening if a woman lies back during labour.

The joints in between the bones of the baby's skull are also flexible, although they fuse later on, and can overlap to help the head fit through the pelvis. By remaining upright a woman can make the most of her pelvis's potential for expansion and assist her baby to be born.

THE WORK OF THE UTERUS

The uterus is a remarkable muscular organ within which the baby grows during pregnancy.

When labour starts the uterus begins to contract and the cervix (or opening) gradually draws up and opens to allow the baby to pass through (see pages 82 and 83). When the mother is upright the baby's head presses on the dilating cervix, thanks again to the effects of the downward force of gravity, and this pressure helps the cervix to open. For this reason studies show that labour tends to be shorter and the contractions more effective when birth is active.

Each time the uterus contracts it tilts forward. If the mother is leaning forward her posture assists the work of the uterus, whereas if she lies back the uterus has to work against the resistance of the pull of gravity. This will make the contractions less effective and the labour far more painful. Any muscle working against resistance soon starts to hurt.

Many women who have given birth actively have told me that the most painful part of the birth was when they had to lie down to be examined. A woman lying down for birth is, therefore, far more likely to need analgesics.

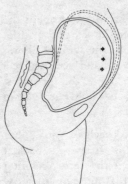

The uterus tilts forward as it contracts

*Lying back the uterus works against
the downwards force of gravity*

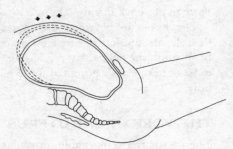

*In an upright position such as standing, squatting or
kneeling gravity assists the whole of the uterus*

CIRCULATION

During pregnancy and birth the baby in the uterus is completely
dependant on the mother's bloodstream for food, oxygen and the
elimination of waste. When a woman lies back the heavy uterus
presses against the major blood vessels (the aorta and the inferior

vena cava) which run along the inside of her spine. This has the effect of slowing down her circulation and reduces the flow of blood to and from the uterus and thus the baby. A baby deprived of oxygen is far more likely to become distressed. For this reason the reclining position is the one most likely to induce foetal distress. The uterus will also function less effectively if circulation is reduced.

HORMONES

The whole process of conceiving, giving birth and nurturing a child is triggered off by the secretion of hormones which act as messengers in the mother's body. If she lies back during labour she is more likely to experience fear, pain and stress. Her body will then secrete stress hormones (such as adrenalin) which actually inhibit the progress of the labour.

We can safely conclude that either lying down or semi-reclining completely disturbs the natural physiology of birth. If the mother is undisturbed and has the freedom of her own body she can use her own instincts to give birth to her baby. Her body is ideally designed for the job and she is the one who knows best how to do it!

2 Pregnancy

Conception and the baby's development in the womb

Pregnancy begins at the moment of conception. One of the millions of sperm that enter the uterus after lovemaking manages to travel down one of the uterine tubes, meets up with a newly erupted ovum and penetrates the outer layers to fertilize the egg.

For the next eight days the fertilized ovum undergoes rapid growth, while spinning down the fallopian tube towards the uterus. By the time it arrives it is a cluster of cells shaped rather like a mulberry. It usually lands near the top of the uterus and from there sends tiny blood vessels into the blood-rich uterine wall. These are the early beginnings of the baby's placenta. In the weeks that follow the cells differentiate and separate into those that form the foetus, those that form the sac of membranes which surround and protect it and those that make up the umbilical cord and placenta.

By the end of the third month the baby is perfectly formed and lies protected within the uterus, floating in the amniotic fluid which surrounds it throughout pregnancy. In the following six months both the uterus and the baby will grow larger until, at term the uterus comes right up to your partner's ribs and the baby inside her weighs an average of 6–8 lb and floats in about 10 pints of amniotic fluid.

The *uterus* is about 4 inches long before pregnancy and shaped rather like a pear. It lies deep within the pelvis, between the bladder in front and the lower part of the bowel and rectum behind. As the baby develops the uterus grows right up out of the pelvis, until, at term (as just mentioned) it fills almost the entire abdomen.

The top part of the uterus is called the *fundus* and the lower part,

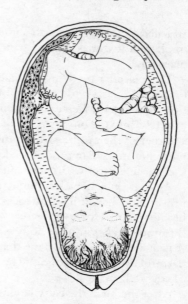

Baby in the womb surrounded by waters and
membranes with cord and placenta

the neck or opening, is called the *cervix*. The cervix lies at the top of
the vagina and is normally tightly closed. It is a circular sphincter in
shape. During pregnancy it is sealed with a plug of jelly, like
mucus, which forms a protective barrier. This comes away when
the birth is imminent or during labour when the cervix becomes
thinner and then slowly dilates or opens to allow the baby to pass
through.

During the first stage of labour the uterus contracts rhythmically
to open at its base, and then once it is open in the second stage it
contracts powerfully from the top to expel the baby. After the birth,
it will contract each time the baby suckles and eventually return to its
previous size and shape within the pelvis.

The membranes which line the inside of the womb form a bag
which surrounds the baby and contains the amniotic fluid. These
protect him from infection and usually remain intact throughout the
pregnancy. Just before or during the labour they will burst open and
release some or all of the amniotic fluid.

The *placenta* is made up of a network of blood vessels which, when
spread out, resemble the roots of a tree. They are held together by a
membrane. At delivery the placenta looks like a large piece of liver
and is about a third of the size of the baby. The placenta is usually

attached to the uterine wall somewhere at the top end, unless it has implanted lower down, in which case it is known as a low-lying placenta.

The placenta performs a vital function during pregnancy for it breathes, digests and excretes for the baby in the womb. It is here that the baby receives its nourishment and passes back waste products into the bloodstream of the mother. The baby's circulation and that of the mother are completely separate and the exchange of nutrients and waste products takes place where the blood vessels of the placenta meet with those of the uterine wall.

At one time it was thought that the placenta acted as a filter, preventing harmful substances from crossing into the baby's bloodstream. However, research has shown that almost anything the mother takes into her body will pass through to the baby. For this reason it is very important that the mother eats well and avoids harmful drugs and alcohol. (The occasional glass of wine is all right, of course.)

After the birth the baby begins to breathe independently through its lungs and establishes contact with the mother's breast. The uterus contracts strongly causing the placenta to separate from its walls. Further contractions expel the placenta and the bag of membranes (known as the afterbirth).

The blood vessels of the placenta unite in the middle to form three large blood vessels which intertwine to create the *umbilical cord*. One of these carries fresh blood from the placenta to the baby and the other two carry blood containing waste products from the baby back to the placenta. The umbilical cord is attached to the baby's body at the navel and is his lifeline during the months in the womb. The baby's heart pumps blood through its body which then circulates through the umbilical cord to the placenta and simultaneously through the cord again back to the baby.

The umbilical cord pulsates constantly and continues to function for some minutes after the birth until the baby has made the transition to breathing through his own lungs for the first time. Only when the function of the placenta has ceased does it separate from the wall of the uterus, nature providing the baby with a double life-line while the transition to independence takes place. This is why it is important not to sever the link and cut the cord prematurely, while it is still pulsating and before it has ceased to be useful. Many birth attendants have been trained to cut the cord immediately after birth, so this is a point worth discussing with them beforehand (see page 110).

As the baby grows and develops your partner will begin to feel movement within her body, first noticeable around the end of the fourth or beginning of the fifth month. You should also be able to feel the baby moving inside by holding your hands against her abdomen a few weeks later. In the months that follow the baby's movements will become more noticeable until, by the end of pregnancy you will literally see the outline of the belly change shape as the baby moves.

Researchers believe that the unborn child is highly sensitive, responding to sound, the emotional state of the mother and touch. * If you feel like it, do not hesitate to talk to, sing to or caress your child in the womb. Small children instinctively do this to their unborn siblings!

The end of the pregnancy

ENGAGEMENT

Towards the end of the pregnancy as the baby grows, his head, being the heaviest part of his body, tends to come down and rest in the lower part of the uterus. This happens some time in the last six to eight weeks in the case of a first birth but is normally closer to the birth or even occurs during labour with subsequent babies. The head usually settles into the brim of the pelvis in readiness for the birth, a process known as 'engagement'. If the baby's head has 'engaged' it is a welcome sign that the birth is likely to be uncomplicated. If it has not, however, this does not necessarily mean that there is any problem, although it may be an indication of one. Sometimes the head does not engage until labour starts even with a first birth.

Once the baby's head engages the mother often experiences a sense of relief and lightening as the baby 'drops'. Often this 'dropping' is visibly noticeable and the whole belly looks lower. Women sometimes experience quite strong contractions in the last few weeks as the uterus prepares for birth. These practice contractions are painless and can last for several minutes, the whole belly going firm and hard until they pass. These are not early labour contractions

---

* *The Secret Life of the Unborn Child*, Dr Thomas Verney with John Kelly, Sphere, 1983

which are much shorter. They are an encouraging sign that all is going as it should be. Occasionally the mother will feel some really strong contractions as the baby's head engages and it is easy to confuse these with the onset of labour.

PRESENTATION

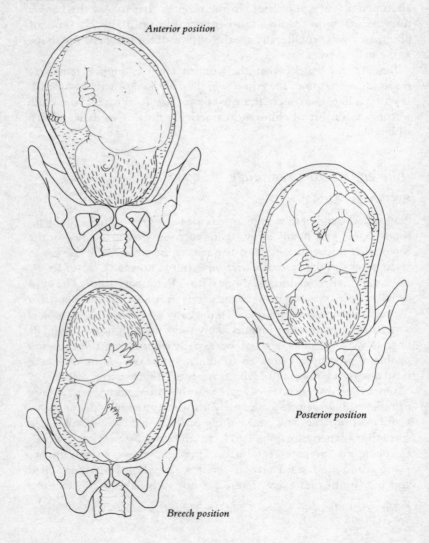

Anterior position

Posterior position

Breech position

The position in which the baby is lying for birth becomes an important issue in the final weeks and regular stretching during pregnancy (see Chapter 3) will help to ensure that the baby settles into the right position for birth.

Anterior position

The majority of babies lie in what is known as the anterior position, i.e. head down with the body flexed, the limbs facing inwards towards the mother's spine and his own spine against the mother's abdominal wall, usually a little to the left or right of her navel. This is the best position for an easy passage through the birth canal.

Posterior position

Here the baby also lies head down but the other way round so that his limbs face towards the mother's abdominal wall and his spine lies against hers. This position is a variation of the normal one and can sometimes be a little more difficult, resulting in a longer first stage and more backache for the mother as the back of the baby's head presses against her cervix.

It often happens that the head will rotate of its own accord into the anterior position during the labour. When the birth is active it is much easier to cope with a posterior position and the necessity for forceps is less likely (see page 89).

Breech position

The baby lies with his head upwards and his bottom or feet above the cervix. From a mechanical point of view this presents certain difficulties as the head, being the largest part of its body, comes out last. This means that the umbilical cord is delivered before the head and if the birth of the head is slow there is a greater risk of compression of the cord or of the premature separation of the placenta. These risks are increased if the mother lies down and does not have the help of gravity or the maximum opening of her pelvis. For this reason, when birth is supine breech babies are often delivered by forceps or Caesarean section and usually in hospital. If, however, a breech birth is active and the mother assumes a supported standing squat position most breech births are uncomplicated and can be seen as variations of the normal.

At the time of writing very few obstetricians and midwives have tried or will consider delivering a breech baby this way, but in some hospitals – such as Michel Odent's in Pithiviers, France, where they have long experience of active birth – it is quite normal for such a birth to be active and spontaneous. Their statistics show that there is no increased risk in allowing breech birth to be natural, in fact the risks seem to be reduced.

Try this

If the baby is lying breech in the eighth month (i.e. four weeks before the birth) the mother can try the following exercise. Research has shown that over 80 per cent of breech babies turn spontaneously if this exercise is kept up persistently.

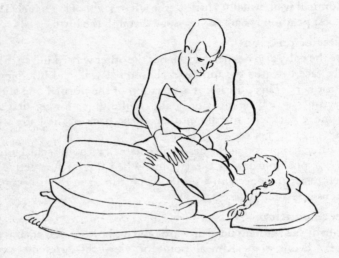

Before she starts she should ask the midwife to show her exactly how the baby is lying so that she can tell where the head is and how the body is positioned. Then she should lie on her back on the floor, placing three firm cushions under her buttocks so that her hips are raised higher than her head. In this position she should massage her belly (you can help) in the direction in which she would like the baby to turn. She should try to communicate with the baby through concentration and gentle touch and continue for ten minutes. The exercise should be repeated several times during the day.

Once your partner suspects that the baby has moved she should stop the exercise and check as soon as possible with her doctor or midwife whether this is the case. If the baby has turned she should then start squatting a lot to encourage the head to engage. This exercise can take several weeks to work and perserverance is the answer. I know of one baby which suddenly turned four days after the expected due date!

When trying to turn a breech baby homoeopaths recommend that the mother takes a dose of the homoeopathic remedy Pulsatilla 200X. For those who use homoeopathics this may be helpful in addition to the exercise.

Transverse position
Very rarely a baby lies in a transverse position with his body across the lower part of the uterus. Unless the baby moves down of its own accord help will be needed for delivery.

You and your partner during pregnancy

The nine months of a pregnancy are usually divided into three trimesters. During the first three months the pregnancy is being established and the mother will see no obvious visible sign of any change in the shape of her belly. Her body is accepting and adjusting to the implantation of the foetus in the uterus. Simultaneously the foetus is undergoing rapid growth and development. This is a vital time for the baby when his body and organic systems are being formed. Many women feel the same as usual or even exceptionally well at this time. However, some women find the first three months difficult as the hormonal balance of the body changes and they settle into the pregnancy. Morning sickness and tiredness are very common.

This can often be a time of emotional turmoil. For most women the psychological adjustment to the fact they are having a baby and becoming a mother needs getting used to! Pregnancy is a time of growth and change for all members of the family and as the father you too can experience an upheaval at this time as your new responsibilities and the changing situation become a reality. Somehow this is accepted in the mother-to-be but all too often the father is simply relied upon for his support and understanding. It is important to realize that these nine months are a period of preparation and growth for you too.

It helps if you share your feelings and talk openly with your partner and with other fathers. If there is a birth preparation course for couples in your area you will probably enjoy meeting other men who are also entering into fatherhood for the first time.

In the second trimester (three to six months) things usually settle down. Many women enjoy this period and feel radiantly well and fitter than ever before.

The last three months, as the time of birth gets closer, can also be quite turbulent emotionally. Your partner may feel less comfortable physically as the baby reaches full size. Sometimes these last few weeks can seem to last an eternity as everyone focuses on the coming event and excitement and tension mount. The mother is likely to experience rapid changes of mood and it is important to make a special effort to be sensitive to each other and spend time together, stretching and massaging (see chapters 3 and 4), going for walks and doing things you enjoy, as your sense of becoming a family grows.

NUTRITION

Eating well in pregnancy is very important, both for the mother and the baby developing inside her and a good diet can go a long way to eliminate complications during pregnancy and birth.

During pregnancy a woman needs 30 per cent more protein and vitamins than usual and extra iron and supplementary vitamins are often recommended. She also needs to drink a little more than usual: about 3 quarts of liquid a day. Whatever your diet, whether you eat meat, fish, eggs, cheese and dairy products, are vegetarian or eat macrobiotic foods, make sure that your partner takes enough protein and try to include whole grains rather than refined wherever possible, i.e. wholemeal bread rather than white, brown rice and wholewheat pasta. It is important that she has plenty of fresh fruit and vegetables, especially leafy green vegetables and a calcium food such as milk, cheese, yoghurt or cottage cheese.

Pregnant women often crave certain tastes and foods. These cravings should be taken seriously as very often her body will be her best guide as to what she needs. Watch out however, for an excessive indulgence in carbohydrates! It is a good idea to keep a supply of nutritious but unstarchy snack foods such as nuts and raisins, carrots, celery and so on within easy reach!

For those who prefer a homoeopathic programme, tissue salts can be taken instead of supplementary vitamins and iron. The following programme is recommended for pregnancy:

2nd and 6th month: CALC FLUOR 6X + MAG PHOS 6X + FERR PHOS 6X
3rd and 7th month: CALC FLUOR 6X + MAG PHOS 6X + NAT MUR 6X
4th and 8th month: CALC FLUOR 6X + NAT MUR 6X + SILICA 6X
5th and 9th month: CALC FLUOR 6X + FERR PHOS 6X + SILICA 6X

These are available from good homoeopathic pharmacies.

LOVEMAKING

There are many old-fashioned taboos and old wives' tales about this subject, but in fact it is perfectly safe to make love during pregnancy. The only good medical reasons to abstain from intercourse are if your partner has had a previous miscarriage or some bleeding and is concerned in the early weeks that she may lose the baby, or if she has had a problem with previous premature births.

There is nothing wrong with making love right up until the actual birth. In fact this is often a very good way to encourage labour to start as semen contains prostoglandin, a hormone which causes the cervix to soften to allow the sperm to enter the womb. However, you will probably find that there are times when your partner is less interested in lovemaking than normally, or she may be more interested than ever. You too are likely to have changing feelings: this is quite normal.

When making love experiment with different positions such as with your partner on top or sideways with her in front of you. Many people refrain from lovemaking because they are concerned that the baby could be damaged in some way. There is no need to be worried about this and in fact the baby probably benefits from the release of pleasant and orgasmic feelings and your closeness. Some couples enjoy a new freedom in their lovemaking as at this time they need have no inhibitions about the woman becoming pregnant! So, far from limiting your sex life pregnancy provides a good opportunity for you to use your imagination and to experiment and explore different ways of showing your care and affection for each other.

THE MINOR DISCOMFORTS OF PREGNANCY

Your partner is likely to be feeling and looking very well during these nine months, particularly if she is stretching regularly. However, there are some very common discomforts that can arise and usually there is a way in which you can help. They are listed below alphabetically for easy reference.

Backache

Make sure you do a stretching session together every day, (see Chapter 3), paying particular attention to the instructions to keep the spine straight.

If your partner has pain in her lower back or indeed if you do yourself, add these two exercises to your routine.

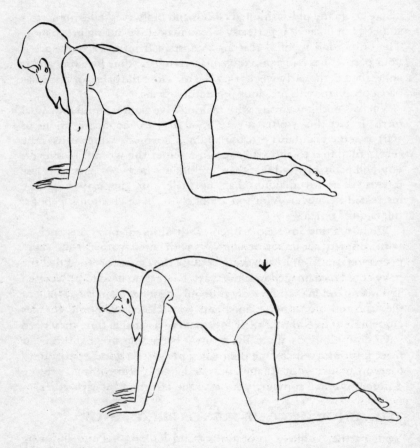

1   Kneel on your hands and knees in the all-fours position on the floor. Tighten your buttocks and tuck in your pelvis so that your back rounds like a cat arching its back. Hold for a few seconds then let go. Repeat ten times.

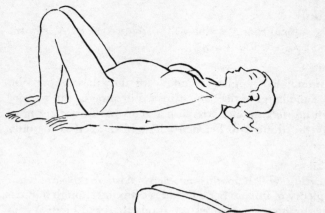

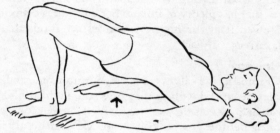

2   Lie on your back on the floor. Bend your knees and bring your
    feet in close to your buttocks keeping the soles on the floor. Put
    your arms by your sides with hands palms down on the ground.
    Tighten your buttocks and, pressing your heels into the ground,
    lift up your pelvis as high as you comfortably can. Hold for a few
    seconds and then let go. Repeat ten times.

These two exercises strengthen the buttock muscles which give
support to the lower back and correct the tilt of the pelvis.
    Try massaging your partner's lower back (see page 77) after the
exercises.

Breasts
Your partner's breasts may become tender and enlarged during
pregnancy. Suggest that she gets a good supporting bra and be
sensitive when touching her. During pregnancy her breasts may
begin to produce a yellowish fluid called colostrum which is the
highly nutritious first milk for the baby.

Bleeding gums

Caused by hormonal changes, this will stop once the baby is born. She could use a softer toothbrush!

Breathlessness

This is common in late pregnancy and is caused by the compression of the ribcage and lungs as the baby grows. Encourage your partner to relax with her feet up and stretch her arms back over her head while slowly breathing into her belly. The birth itself is the only lasting remedy.

Constipation

Lots of squatting will help this problem. Also make sure your partner has plenty of fibre in her diet and is drinking enough liquids. Stewed fruit, bran, and tomatoes are foods that will help. Avoid laxatives.

Cramps

Cramps in the calves are very common and can be quite alarming if they occur suddenly as they often do, in the middle of the night. You can help by getting your partner to bend her foot, extend her heel and bring her toes towards her head. Massage gently until the pain goes. Suggest that she do the calf stretch (see page 65) before going to bed.

Dizziness

This is caused by the secretion of hormones which can soften all the blood vessels and slow your partner's circulation. Suggest that she change positions slowly and eat small meals frequently rather than three big meals a day to keep up her blood sugar level.

Haemorrhoids

The best remedy for this complaint is to tighten and release the anal muscles fifty times before getting up in the morning and before going to sleep at night. With perseverance it is possible to cure the condition.

Heartburn

This very common and uncomfortable complaint is caused by hormones softening the valve between the stomach and the oesophagus. Suggest your partner takes small meals frequently rather than large ones and avoids foods which make it worse.

Some women swear that a juice made from three umeboshi plums boiled in a saucepan of water works wonders. The plums are available from health food stores. Keep the juice in the fridge and sip when necessary. Soy sauce can be added for taste as they are very sour.

Insomnia

This is common too. Your partner may be worrying about something, so encourage her to share her feelings. She may just be uncomfortable! Hot milk, a sense of humour and a cuddle can solve the problem. You can always reassure her that if the body rests we don't need all that much sleep and that probably if she stops worrying about it she will sleep better. Camomile tea before retiring has a soporific effect and glass of wine with dinner may help. A good supply of pillows might make her more comfortable.

Morning sickness

This can be caused by hormonal changes or alternatively be a physical and emotional reaction to being pregnant. It tends to occur mainly in the first three months although some women suffer from nausea and loss of appetite throughout pregnancy. If the problem is severe I suggest consulting a homoeopath as there are several helpful remedies. Tea and crackers before getting out of bed in the morning may help. Sometimes the period of feeling sick can be in the evening or afternoon rather than the morning. Extra Vitamin B complex may help.

Sciatica

Sciatica is a sudden shooting pain down the leg caused by pressure on the sciatic nerve in the area of the sacro–illiac joint. Your partner should do the exercises recommended for backache and concentrate on Japanese sitting and the spinal stretch (see pages 58 and 68). Suggest that she lie on her side and then you can gently rub her lower back until it passes.

Stretch marks

These are red striations or lines which come up, usually on the breasts, thighs, belly or hips. Stretching helps to prevent them as does firm massage. If your partner already has some stretch marks, suggest that she massages them with Vitamin E oil. After the birth they will become much lighter losing the red colour and continuing with Vitamin E can eventually almost remove them.

Swelling – oedema

This occurs most often in the fingers, ankles and knees and is caused by fluid retention. It can be helped by homoeopathic treatment and is nothing to worry about unless it is combined with other symptoms such as a rise in blood pressure and protein in the urine. However it should be checked by the midwife or doctor who will probably recommend that your partner eliminates salt from her diet.

Tiredness
A pregnant woman needs plenty of rest. Regular stretching, combined with enough rest will help to prevent fatigue. Make sure her diet is good too.

Urinary frequency
This is caused in the early months by hormones and towards the end of pregnancy by pressure from the uterus on the bladder. Don't be surprised if your partner is up several times in the night towards the end.

3 Exercise

Working on your body

We are all born completely supple. A young child can make any of the movements suggested in this chapter with ease and everyone can squat before they stand up. Indeed, this is a resting position for the body and in countries where people squat habitually, they will sit, work and rest in this position for hours. Poor physical education in schools and bad habits such as sitting in chairs, always taking the car instead of walking, wearing high heels or tight shoes takes its toll on us by reducing our need and capacity to use our bodies as nature intended. The result is that we do not make the full range of movements which we are capable of and our joints and muscles become stiff.

Stiffness and tension in the body are also caused by suppressed feelings and emotions. The catastrophic situations, traumas and pain which occur in our lives all cause us to develop a kind of defensive physical armour.

By working on our bodies and releasing stiffness and tension we can free ourselves of pent-up emotions, fear and suppressed feelings in a gradual and gentle way. In our society physical stiffness has reached epidemic proportions without our being aware of it. Very few people have retained the original suppleness of their bodies and most of us are functioning at far less than our full potential. However, we can improve the situation. A stiff muscle can regain its elasticity and the movement of a joint can increase significantly with exercise.

43

Stretching together

You and your partner have a marvellous opportunity during the months of pregnancy to work together, not only to prepare for the birth but also to benefit yourselves. Indeed, pregnancy can be a time of growth and transformation for the whole family.

As the baby develops within the womb the mother too is blossoming into a new phase of her life. Her body has a natural tendency towards health and vitality. She should make the most of this opportunity to become more relaxed and supple so as to be at her best for birth and motherhood. As her partner you can join her in a daily session of stretching together and enjoy the benefits of improving your physical health and discovering a new way to relax. Spending time together in this way will create a closeness and harmony between you which can continue into labour, birth and parenthood itself.

During labour you will find that simply physically supporting a woman giving birth requires quite a lot of stamina and strength so now is the time that you should loosen up stiff knees and ankles and learn to relax. If you yourself can develop ease, comfort and familiarity with the supporting positions you may use during labour and birth you will be able to help your partner considerably to surrender to the powerful forces working within her body. Stretching brings you directly in touch with your body and is a fundamental way of releasing tension in your muscles and joints. With regular practice your body becomes more supple and your health and vitality improve. Your contact with your partner will deepen. Being more in touch with yourself brings you close to those around you.

Your first relationship with your newborn child will primarily be one of body contact and touch. These months of stretching will help to lay the foundation for holding, caressing and playing, all producing an ease in physical contact which is a vital part of being a good parent or companion to a small child.

STRETCHING RELAXES YOU

Stretching is the simplest and most effective way of relaxing your body. For the last few decades many different techniques for relaxation have been used in preparation for childbirth. Stretching gets down to the fundamental stiffness in your muscles and brings about a physical relaxation which can only arise from improved muscle elasticity.

When you lie down and let go of your thoughts and worries, concentrating on your breathing, you will feel rested and relaxed afterwards but you will have done nothing to alter the chronic tension in your body. On the other hand, if you start from the vantage point of your body, gradually stretching and lengthening stiff muscles and increasing the mobility of joints, you will discover a deep and lasting relaxation which increases with practice.

Try this

This exercise will help you understand how stretching works to relax your body. Stand upright with your feet about 6 inches apart and facing forward. Clasp your hands behind your back. Keeping your back and legs perfectly straight, bend forward from the hips until you begin to feel a stretching sensation in the hamstring muscles at the back of your legs. Hold for a few seconds and then come up slowly.

Our full potential for movement when bending forward is to be able to bring the chest down on to the thighs and knees, folding the body in half like a jack-knife. You will probably find that you were able to do far less than this. The pain you felt in your hamstring muscles as you leant forward was caused by stiffness.

STIFFNESS

Muscles work in teams throughout the body. When one set of muscles is lengthening and relaxing, the other is shortening and contracting. When muscles are not used to their full potential for a long period of time they lose this elasticity and shrink, becoming stiff. When you bend forward the hamstring muscles at the back of your legs lengthen and relax. By making this movement regularly the muscles will gradually regain their elasticity, the stiff, painful sensations will ease and become pleasurable and your vital energy will flow more easily.

To sum up:
* Stretching is a passive, non-strenuous form of exercise which effectively releases chronic tension and stiffness in the musculature of your body.

★ It is a system of lengthening and relaxing the muscles and improving the movement of the joints by harnessing the help of the force of gravity.

★ It can be used to great effect by men, women and children alike and will help the athlete, sportsman or businessman as much as the mother about to give birth to a child.

WHY THE PREGNANT WOMAN SHOULD STRETCH

For a pregnant woman stretching is a wonderful preparation for labour and birth. The health and development of her baby depend on her own health. At this time more than any other stretching is invaluable and she will benefit for a host of reasons.

★ Her body has a natural tendency to become more supple in readiness for the birth. Hormones secreted during pregnancy soften her joints, ligaments and muscles making her pelvis more expandable and flexible. By stretching she can take full advantage of nature's preparation to increase her pelvic capacity and to relax and strengthen the muscles and joints of her whole body, but particularly of her pelvis. The fit of her child's head in her pelvis is so exact that the smallest increase of her pelvic opening during labour is significant and beneficial.

★ The stretching exercises help her to become comfortable in positions such as squatting and kneeling which she will find useful for labour and birth.

★ By freeing herself of unnecessary stiffness and tension during pregnancy she will be able to cope better with the pain which is generally inevitable in strong labour. She will learn to go beyond the normal limits and to make friends with her pain.

★ Stretching improves the circulation. A muscle that is supple and elastic allows blood to pass through it freely so that oxygen and waste products are carried efficiently through the body. This is especially important during pregnancy and birth when the developing child in the womb is depending on his mother's circulation for nourishment and the removal of waste.

★ In its turn good circulation improves the flow of lymph through the body and this helps to defend the body against bacteria and viruses.

★ Stretching improves breathing by relaxing the muscles directly involved, thus increasing our thoracic capacity. When we breathe we also depend on the indirect action of our skeletal muscles to pump blood from the limbs up to the heart. So by stretching the whole body we improve our circulation and our breathing and also regulate our blood pressure and heart rate.

* Stretching corrects posture, ensuring that the baby, as it grows, is well supported without strain to the mother. Backache is prevented or improved, cramp and headaches are eased.

* Stretching gives one's body a sense of lightness which pregnant women find very helpful and an aid in eliminating fatigue and giving energy.

* Most importantly, stretching brings the mother deeply in contact with her body. She will discover a new physical intimacy with herself which will lead her to discover her own inner resources for giving birth. By starting with her own body in preparing for birth and motherhood she will automatically discover her deep, instinctive knowledge of birthing and caring for her baby.

As her partner, by stretching together every day you will be helping her in the best possible way.

Getting started

Set aside half an hour or an hour per day, preferably at a time when you will not be disturbed. It is best not to eat just before stretching.

You will need a blanket each or a carpeted room to work in with one wall free.

At first when you start you will become aware of your stiffness. As you begin to use and stretch your muscles you will feel the tightness as a cramp–like pain in the muscles or an aching sensation in the joints. If you persevere for a few days, however, this discomfort will ease as your muscles begin to relax. After a few weeks the stretching sensations will become pleasant and relieving and both you and your partner will begin to feel the benefits.

As you discover your own stiffness you will notice the differences between your body and that of your partner. You may have stiff knees and more flexible hips than her or vice versa. Men are often stiffer than women to start with but if this is the case do not be discouraged as anyone can become more flexible. By allowing her to help you, you are also helping her!

Start each exercise gradually, holding it for only a few seconds to begin with until you can remain comfortably in position for three to five minutes or more. Become familiar and comfortable with each movement first before you attempt the 'partner stretches' as these will help you to go further than your usual limit.

The stretching exercises that follow are intended specifically as basic preparation for birth. The emphasis is therefore on the pelvic area, knees, ankles and parts of the body which are most important for comfort in the positions used by both partners during labour and birth. Also included are some basic stretches for the rest of the body. If, however, you and your partner wish to go further with this system of exercise see Recommended Reading on page 163 for a list of books which are more comprehensive.

Wear loose, comfortable clothing (if any) for these exercises – shorts or a track suit are ideal.

Stretching and breathing exercises

DEEP BREATHING

Before attempting any positional exercises it is important to learn how to breathe correctly. This is deeply relaxing at any time and will be of great value in helping you both to let go of tension while stretching and also for your partner, both during pregnancy and when she is coping with contractions during labour.

Just as most people in our society are physically stiff, so most of us also have incorrect breathing habits. If you observe the breathing of a young child or baby you will soon see that the abdomen moves rhythmically up and down as the child inhales and exhales. By the time most of us reach adulthood we tend to breathe both more shallowly into the chest rather than the abdomen and also too fast. Often we are inhaling the next breath before we have emptied our lungs completely of stale air from the last.

Concentration on the rhythm of the breath has great value in that it enables us to become centred more deeply within ourselves. Every form of meditation is based on an awareness of inhalation and exhalation. By spending a few minutes daily on awareness of the breath it is possible to quieten the mind, stop or slow down the internal dialogue that usually spins around our heads and to find an inner peace and relaxation. It is a way of deepening our level of consciousness.

When a woman goes through the hours of labour and her body opens in readiness to give birth to her child, she experiences a profound change from her normal, everyday consciousness. For some women this can be a deeply spiritual and ecstatic experience and indeed for her partner too. On the other hand, if she becomes tense and anxious she may tend to inhale deeply and hold her breath, fighting against what is happening in her body. By practising breathing together you will be able to 'breathe' along with her when she is in labour and this can make all the difference.

1   BREATH AWARENESS

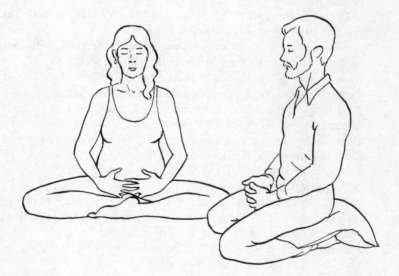

Note
While learning this exercise it is a good idea at first for one of you to read the instructions out aloud slowly while the other does the exercise and then change round until you are both familiar with it.

The cycle of the breath

a)   Seat yourself comfortably in a quiet place. You can simply sit crosslegged on the floor or else kneel on your haunches, placing a small cushion between your buttocks and your calves. If you like, lean against a wall so that your back is well supported. If neither of these positions is comfortable use a straight-backed chair.

b)   Close your eyes and turn your awareness inwards. Become aware of your spine: a straight line from the top of your head to your tailbone.

c)   Lift your shoulders up towards your ears and then drop them so that they are relaxed.

   Open your chest, bringing your breastbone up and your shoulder blades towards each other at the back.

   Relax your arms, allowing your hands to lie softly in your lap or else palms upwards on your knees.

   Let your head tilt slightly forward, neck relaxed and chin coming down towards the breastbone.

   Allow all the muscles of your face to become soft and expressionless and all tension in your body to melt away.

d)   Now, quietly with your body completely relaxed and comfortable, centre your awareness on the rhythm of your breathing. Notice each breath, each inhalation and each exhalation and continue for a few breaths.

e)   Breathing in and out through your nose, begin to concentrate on the exhalation. Each time you breathe out, empty your lungs completely. Slowly sigh the breath out until you have a feeling of emptiness.

f)   After each exhalation pause for a few seconds, stay with the feeling of emptiness until you feel an urge to breathe in and then allow the inhalation to come of its own accord.

g)   Continue for a moment or two on your own, concentrating on the outbreath, pausing and then inhaling.

Abdominal breathing

a)   Repeat the above exercise until you are breathing comfortably.

b)   Then place your hands on your lower abdomen. Tighten your abdominal muscles a little so that you feel your belly draw inwards away from your hands. Then relax and even push your abdominal muscles out a little, just gently, so that your belly comes towards your hands.

c) Now try to co-ordinate this action with your breathing. It may be a little confusing at first as you may have the habit of breathing into your chest but with a little practice breathing into your belly will come naturally to you again as it did when you were a child.

As you exhale your belly goes inwards, *away from* your hands as if emptying.

As you inhale your belly comes outwards, *towards* your hands as if it were filling up with air.

Make these movements consciously until they become automatic. It may help to make the sound 'aaah' as you breathe out.

d) Continue for a few more breaths, your belly filling as you breathe in and emptying as you breathe out. Then place your hands in your lap. Breath in and out normally, concentrating on the outbreath, and continue for a few minutes or longer if you like, keeping your awareness on the breathing rhythm.

Variation (See below.)

Abdominal breathing for labour
Repeat the first abdominal breathing exercise, stages a–c, only this time breathe *in* through the nose and *out* through the mouth throughout. At the end return to your normal breathing in and out through the nose. Practise this breathing in combination with the labour positions given on page 84.

Some women are quite comfortable breathing only through the nose in labour but most tend to open their mouths as the efforts needed become stronger. So in preparation it is wise to practise a few minutes of exhalation through the mouth. As the cervix opens to allow the baby to pass through the mother will naturally open her mouth and will probably breathe out increasingly vigorously, perhaps letting out quite a lot of sound at the same time. Many women like to sigh the breath out quietly and find it very helpful if their partner breathes out together with them.

Variation just for you
This is not recommended for your partner as she should not lie flat on her back while pregnant. Try doing this exercise lying flat on

your back on the floor, legs comfortably apart and arms loosely by your sides, palms upwards or hands on your belly. Allow your whole body to become heavy and relaxed and then follow the same instructions.

2   THE BUTTERFLY

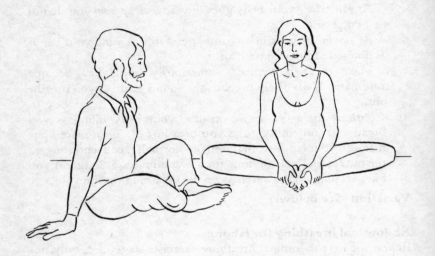

Sit with your back against a wall and legs straight out in front of you. Keeping your spine straight, bring your feet together sole to sole, about 12 inches away from your pubic bone. Clasp your feet with your hands or else place your hands palms down behind you to support your back. Gently work your knees towards the floor, making a bouncing movement, stretching the inside of your thighs and groin. As you begin to loosen up bring your feet in as close as possible to the pubic bone.

Note

Pay special attention to the spine, which must at all times be straight. If the spine collapses, the pelvis tilts backwards and the exercise is of no benefit. If at first you find this exercise difficult, sit on the edge of a small cushion, support your back against a wall or with your hands and gently bounce your knees towards the ground until you begin to loosen up.

Benefits

This exercise lengthens and relaxes the muscles that run along the inside of the thighs and groin and also the pelvic-floor muscles, improving circulation and muscle tone to the whole area. It also corrects the tilt of the mother's pelvis thus ensuring good posture and good support for the growing baby. It helps expand the pelvic canal from side to side increasing the elasticity of the joints.

Partner stretch

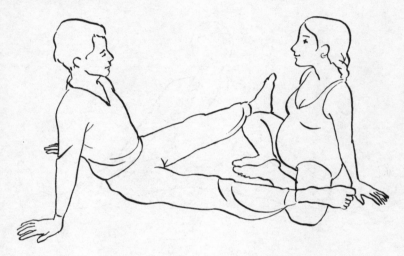

Once you can both comfortably hold this position for five minutes, try doing it with your partner.

When assisting

a) Keep your knees straight and rest your heels on your partner's knees.

b) Support your back with your hands, relax completely and tune into your partner's breathing.

c) The weight of your legs will increase the stretch for your partner. The closer your feet are towards her knees the greater the stretch.

d) Hold for only a second or two the first time, increasing the timing to suit your partner.

When being stretched

a) Keep the back of your pelvis right into the wall and your back straight.

b)   Bring your heels as close as possible to your pubic bone.
c)   Concentrate on your breathing and try to 'let go' and allow your knees to sink slowly to the floor.
d)   Feel the stretch on the inner thighs and groin and let your partner know when you would like to stop.

3   LEGS WIDE APART

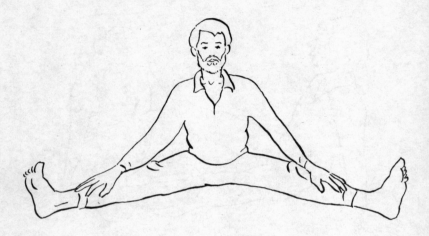

Sit on the floor with your legs wide apart and your back as upright as possible. To keep your back straight sit on the very edge of a small cushion or support yourself by putting your hands on the floor behind you. Tighten your knees and extend your heels, bringing your toes in towards your body. Hold for a few minutes, using your breathing to ease the stretch.

Benefits

This exercise stretches the adductors or inner thigh muscles which are said to be connected with the genital area and uterus. (Reich – psychologist and initiator of Reichian therapy – called them the 'morality muscles'.) Releasing stiffness and tension in this area increases one's enjoyment of sex, allows one to feel more open and also increases vitality and energy. During pregnancy a woman can experience a great improvement in this stretch which will benefit her during labour and birth.

Partner stretch

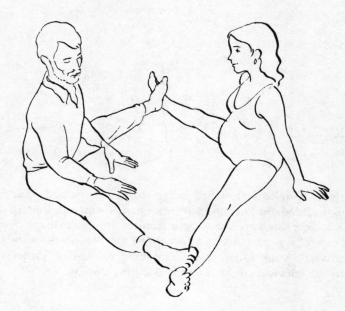

When assisting
a) Keep your knees and back straight, supporting your body by placing your hands on the floor behind you.
b) Place your heels on your partner's ankle bones and gently and very slowly move in closer, spreading her legs further apart until she asks you to stop.
c) Tune into your partner's breathing and directions.
When being stretched
a) Keep your knees and back straight and extend your heels. Keep your body as upright as possible.
b) Tune into your breathing and try to release tension as you breathe out, indicating clearly to your partner how far you would like to be stretched.

4   KNEE STRETCH

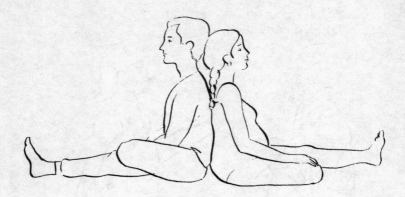

Sit with your legs stretched out in front of you and your back straight. Bend one knee and with your hands bring one foot up on to the opposite thigh as close to your trunk as you can manage. Slowly and carefully work your bent knee down towards the floor and then in towards your other knee. This exercise can be done while watching television or at other times during the day.

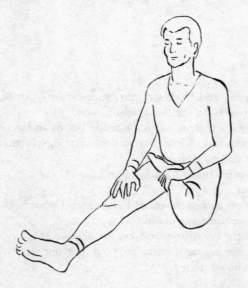

Benefits

The knees are the largest joints in the body and tend to stiffen very easily. To be comfortable in the birth positions and when supporting a woman giving birth actively it is important to work on improving the suppleness of the knees. At first stiff knees are very painful but time and patience will loosen them without force.

5 ANKLE STRETCH

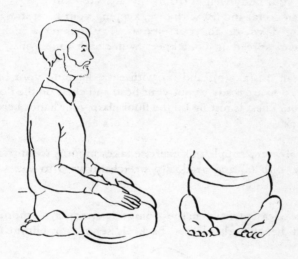

Sit on your heels with your knees together and spine straight. Hold this position for a few minutes. Once you can sit on your heels comfortably, try slowly moving your feet apart and allow your buttocks to touch the floor. Make sure your toes turn inwards and your heels outwards.

Benefits

Many people suffer from stiffness in the knees and ankles and find this exercise very difficult and painful. Regular practice, starting with only a few seconds and building up to five minutes, will increase suppleness in these joints and lessen pain. When starting off or when using this position to help support a woman in labour, try placing a cushion between your buttocks and calves for greater comfort.

6   JAPANESE SITTING

a)   Sit upright with your buttocks between your feet and your knees open as wide as possible, toes pointing inwards towards each other. If you find it difficult to sit between your feet, sit on your heels. Maintain this position for a few seconds, gradually building up to three minutes.

b)   Keeping your back and arms straight, lean forward on to your hands, keeping your buttocks close to your feet. Bend from your hips, not your lower back. Try a rocking movement, shifting your body weight from your arms to your legs.

c)   If you can do (a) and (b) with ease, keeping your back straight, try going down on to your elbows. Try making a rocking movement, spreading your knees wider each time you come forward.

d)   If you can do (a), (b), and (c) with ease, keeping your back straight, you are ready to put your head and chest on the floor. Once your chest is resting on the floor clasp your hands behind your back.

Note

Unless you are very supple this exercise takes months to cultivate. Start slowly with (a) and gradually stretch forward to suit your progress.

Benefits

This exercise releases tension in the groin and pelvic joints, improves posture and benefits the lower back, lessening or eliminating

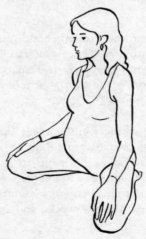

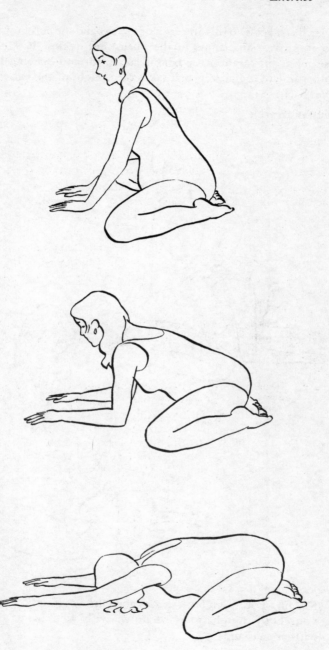

backache and pain in this area. It helps to expand the pelvic outlet and also improves suppleness in the knees and ankles. It is a useful position as preparation for labour and birth and beneficial to the mother in late pregnancy as it takes the weight of the baby off her lower back.

Partner stretch

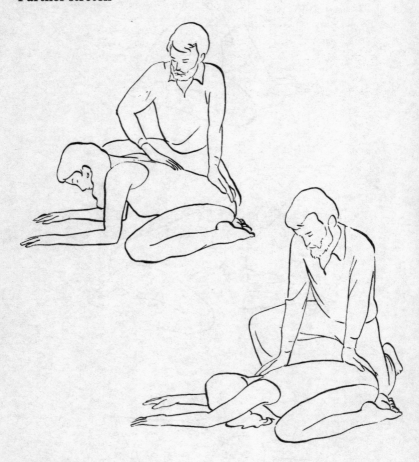

When assisting
a)   Keeping your own back, knees and elbows straight, gently use your body weight to press down with your hands on your partner's sacrum.

b)   Make sure that your partner's spine is straight.
c)   The direction of the weight should be down and back towards
     your partner's feet.
d)   Start gently at first and then if you need to apply more weight do
     so on your partner's exhalation.
e)   Use your body weight and never use force.

When being stretched
a)   Keep your back straight.
b)   Open your knees as wide as possible.
c)   Concentrate on your breathing, particularly the exhalation.

7   SHOULDER STRETCH

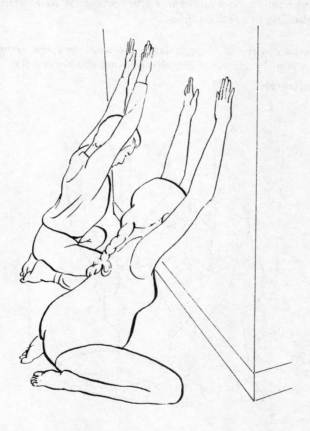

a)   Sit on your heels facing a wall about an arm's length away and spread your knees comfortably apart.

b)   Raise your arms on to the wall, keeping your elbows straight and hands about a shoulder's width apart. Keep your elbows locked straight and your fingers and palms extended to their limits.

c)   Lift your breastbone towards the wall and at the same time drop your shoulders downwards, bringing your shoulder blades together at the back.

d)   You should feel the stretch in your shoulders and arms only. If you feel any discomfort in your back then you need to move a little closer to or further from the wall.

e)   Breathe into it and hold for a few seconds at first, gradually building up to a few minutes.

Benefits

This stretch opens the chest, relaxes the shoulders and arms and improves your breathing, while also relaxing the lower back.

Partner stretch

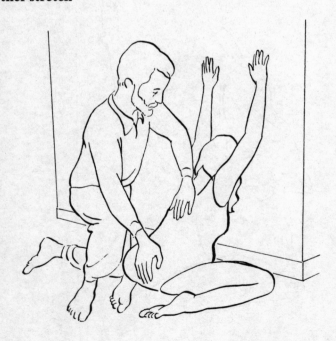

When assisting
a) Keeping your elbows straight, gently lean your body weight downwards and away from your partner's head.
b) The direction of the weight should be down the spine towards the tailbone.
c) Apply your weight gradually, using the heel of your hand for contact with your partner's spine.
d) Tune into your partner's breathing and be guided by his or her instructions.

When being stretched
a) Keep your hands a shoulder's width apart and your elbows straight.
b) Drop your shoulders, bring your chestbone towards the wall and draw your shoulder blades together and down towards your lower back.
c) Make sure you are comfortable and feeling the stretch in the shoulders and arms. Direct your partner so that that the weight of the push is gradual and downwards and you feel the weight leaning on you rather than a pushing pressure.
d) Make sure your partner is not leaning too heavily on your lower back. Most of the emphasis should be on the upper part of the spine around the shoulders.

8 NECK STRETCH

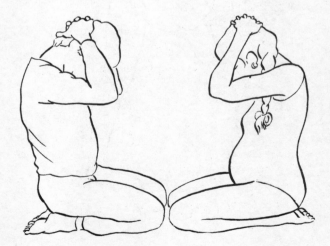

Stand or sit and interlock your hands on the back of your head just beneath your crown. Allow your arms to hang and consciously bring your shoulders and shoulder blades downwards. You should feel the stretch along the back of the neck from the base of the skull to the shoulder blades. Breathe deeply and hold for a few seconds to a minute.

Benefits

This stretch relaxes the muscles of the neck, eyes and face and relieves tension headaches.

9   FORWARD BEND

Stand with your feet slightly apart. Turn your toes in slightly and your heels out. Bend forward from the hips, keeping your spine straight, and clasp your hands behind your back. Hang for a few seconds, breathing deeply. Come up slowly from the hips. Repeat a few times.

Then try this stretch with your feet 3 feet apart.

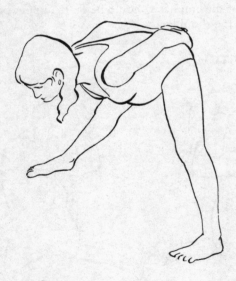

A comfortable way to assist your partner to bend forward in the later months of pregnancy is to stand in front of her and support her weight by holding her elbows. She should keep her back straight in line with her head and arms.

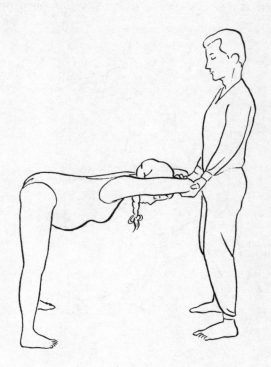

Note
It is important to keep the spine completely straight when doing this exercise and not to bend your back.
Benefits
This exercise stretches the hamstring muscles at the back of the legs, improves circulation and helps to give one energy and reduce fatigue. Most importantly supple hamstrings prevent strain on the lower back and hence backache and bad posture.

10 CALF STRETCH

Stand facing a wall with one leg forward and one back, both feet straight and at right angles to the wall. Lean on to the wall with your elbows, supporting your weight and keeping your hands clasped. Rest your head comfortably on your arms. Bend the front knee and tighten and extend the back knee, pushing your back heel down so

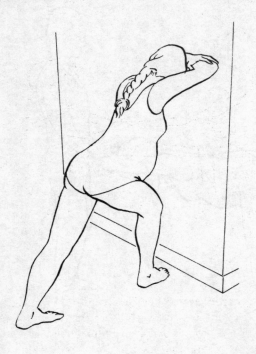

that all the weight of your body is on the back heel. Keep the toes of both feet pointing forwards, angling your back foot to stretch your calf muscles and Achilles tendon. Hold for a few seconds, breathing deeply and then change legs. Repeat several times.

Benefits

This exercise stretches, lengthens and relaxes the calf muscles which increases the flexibility of the ankles and improves squatting. Try alternating this stretch with squatting (Exercise 11), doing a few minutes of each.

11 SQUATTING

a) Stand facing your partner and, keeping elbows straight, clasp each other's arms above the elbow. Keep your feet about 12 inches apart with your toes pointing straight forward to start with.

b) Pulling on each other for support and balance, squat down slowly together, turning your feet out slightly and finding the

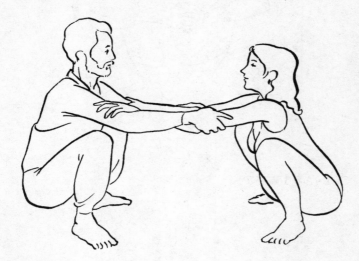

right distance from each other for a comfortable balance. Spread your knees as wide as you can and keep the weight of your body on the outside of your feet, lifting your arches. Hold for a few seconds at first, building up to three to five minutes. Try alternating this exercise with the calf stretch (Exercise 10).

c) Practise this exercise for a few minutes daily with your partner and also encourage her to squat on a low stool or pile of books instead of sitting on a chair.

Benefits

This is the most important of all the exercises as it is the ideal physiological posture for birth and pregnancy and helps to expand and relax the pelvis in the best possible way. In this position the pelvis is at its most open and the soft tissues of the pelvic area are completely relaxed.

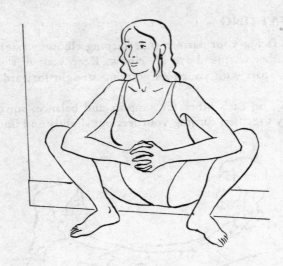

12   SPINAL TWIST

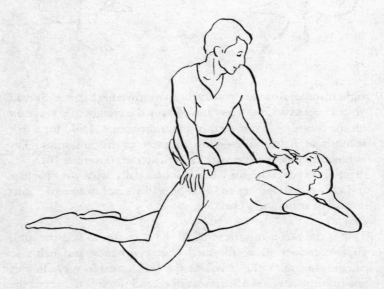

Lie on your back with your hands interlocked underneath your head and elbows flat on the floor. Bend your knees keeping your feet on the floor. Cross one leg over the other and hold the foot of the top leg under the calf of the lower leg. Keeping your shoulders and both elbows on the floor, rotate your pelvis, bringing your top knee down to its opposite side. Hold for a few seconds, breathing deeply, and then repeat on the other side. Increase gradually to one minute or more on each side.

Benefits

This stretch is deeply relaxing to the whole body and benefits the spine, rotating and lubricating the joints between the vertebrae. It helps and prevents backache and stretches the muscles on the side of your trunk and the upper chest.

Partner stretch

When assisting

a) Use your foot to anchor your partner's elbow firmly and gently to the floor. If your partner cannot do this, suggest that she put the arm down by her side and put your weight on the shoulder instead.

b) Put one hand on your partner's knee and the other at the back of the hips.

c) Lean your body weight slowly on to your partner's knee and at the same time, with a gentle and even force, rotate your partner's hips.

d) Tune into your partner's response and breathing.

e) Repeat on the other side.

When being stretched

a) Breathe deeply and make sure you are completely passive and relaxed.

b) Guide your partner by explaining what you are feeling, whether you want more or less weight or whether you want the stretch held at a particular point.

13   RESTING

At the end of a stretching session spend a few minutes resting. You can lie flat on your back on the floor. Your partner should lie on her side with her head and right knee comfortably supported with pillows.

Sport and other forms of exercise

If your partner is accustomed to playing tennis, jogging or cycling, it is possible to continue during pregnancy provided that she is moderate and adapts to the advancing pregnancy as her body dictates. Beneficial exercise ideal for pregnancy is walking and swimming.

4 Massage

Touch is our first sensation. The embryo in the womb will feel through its skin before the eyes and ears have even begun to develop. Our skin is the oldest and most sensitive of our organs.

How we touch ourselves, each other and the world around us is of great importance to our general health and wellbeing. It is the way we comfort and caress one another and express our love and affection. Similarly touching is the most basic means of communication between mother, father and newborn baby. The way in which babies are handled is therefore of prime importance for their healthy physical and behavioural development. Body contact and comfort are fundamental to our ability to love one another.

In his book *Touching* Ashley Montague has collected much research on the subject and draws the following conclusion: 'It is evident that in mammals generally continuous stimulation is important at all stages of development, but particularly important during the early days of the life of the newborn, during pregnancy, delivery and during the nursing period.' This may seem to be stating the obvious. Many of us, however, have grown up today in a world in which mothers and babies have been separated at birth and where we have literally lost touch both with ourselves and each other.

Partnering a woman through pregnancy, birth and motherhood is a perfect opportunity to regain our skills in the way we touch one another. Being massaged is not only very comforting during pregnancy, but for many women it is one of the most helpful ways to cope with labour as well as being vital preparation for motherhood. By learning how to touch yourselves and each other you will discover a wonderful language, a new way to communicate and share your energy.

The aim of massage is to stimulate the soft tissues of the body. This stimulation can be light or deep depending on what is needed. It will assist blood circulation and increase the suppleness and relaxation of the tissues.

Before beginning to massage your partner it is a good idea to work on your own body, to experiment and explore the skin, muscles, bones, and joints. When you begin to feel confident, then try working together.

Massage is essentially an intuitive exploration and the instructions given below are intended as a guide to get you started. Once you relax and become creative you will discover your own natural way of touching and the special needs, likes and dislikes of your partner.

There are many ways in which we can touch one another.

SURFACE STROKING

The flat of the hand is used to stroke the skin gently with a light but firm pressure. In severe pain or spasm this very light stroking is often the only form of massage possible.

KNEADING

This form of massage goes deeper and works the muscles by alternately squeezing and releasing them in the same way as we knead dough when making bread.

DEEP PRESSURE

With deep pressure you work on the bones rather than the muscles and the skin, using your thumb, fingers or the heel of your hand to exert quite a lot of pressure according to your partner's needs.

PRESSURE-POINT MASSAGE

As you get to know your own body and that of your partner you will discover certain painful spots. With pressure–point massage you use a deeper penetration to exert pressure on these spots, making small circular movements, usually with your thumbs. You will feel either a hard, tense muscle or small, crystal–like grains close to the bones. By applying quite strong pressure and movement to these areas you can gradually massage away the tension and pain.

RELAX YOUR HANDS

Before beginning to massage spend five minutes warming and loosening your hands. Hold each movement for five to ten seconds.

a) Hold your thumb close to the nail between your fingers and twist and rotate it to its limit in both directions.

b) In the same way rotate each finger to its limit in both directions.

c) Flex or bend *forward* each of the knuckle joints in turn.

d) Repeat with the middle joint of each finger and then the top finger joint.

e) Bend your wrist and thumb downwards towards your lower arm.

f) Now extend or bend *backwards* each of your fingers in turn, extending all three of your finger joints to their limits.

g) Shake your whole hand vigorously from the wrist allowing the arm to hang loosely from the shoulder.

FOOT MASSAGE

a) Sit on the floor or on a chair in a comfortable position, bringing one foot close to your body. If you like you could use a little warm vegetable oil such as olive or almond and start by using the flat of your hand and stroking your skin, spreading the oil over the whole foot and the calf.

b) Next bend all the toes forwards and then backwards Squeeze the whole foot firmly in your hand, passing down the sole to the heel and then up the muscles at the back of the calf. Keep up these squeezing movements and come down the front of the calf and the top part of the foot.

c) Now twist and rotate each of the toes to their limit in both directions and then bend each toe forwards at the knuckle joint and then backwards in turn.

d) Now begin to go a little deeper, using your thumbs to exert more pressure, and slowly explore the bones of the foot starting under the big toe and passing down the instep to the ankle and Achilles tendon, continuing until the whole foot including the calves has been worked. Along the way you will probably find many painful spots and you can linger here a while massaging away the tension.

e) Finish by rotating the whole foot at the ankle joint and stroking the surface of the skin.

f)   When you feel confident enough to start with your partner, make sure she is comfortable. She could sit against a pile of cushions with head and body completely supported and legs gently apart. You can then sit crosslegged in front of her, holding the foot you are working on in your lap.

FACE AND HEAD MASSAGE

Sit comfortably on a chair or on the floor.

a)   Using your fingertips start off by smoothing away all tension on your forehead, working from the middle outwards.

b)   Next, using your thumbs and exerting as much pressure as you want, make small, circular movements all along the top of the eyebrows. Start from the nose and work along the bony rim of the eye socket and then the lower rim.

c)   Next, massage the bony part of the nose, bending the tip first to the left and then to the right.

d)   Now massage the cheekbones starting with a firm, smooth stroke from the nose and working towards the temples.

e)   Using your fingertips, massage the upper jaw concentrating on the corners of the jaw, where tension tends to accumulate, and passing along the gums and teeth above the mouth.

f)   Massage the lower jaw, pressing firmly into the jawbone.

g)   Continue in this way to the temples, ears, the base of the skull, the back of the neck, and shoulders.

h)   Finally massage the scalp and end by smoothly stroking the whole face from the centre outwards.

i)   Place your fingertips over the eyeballs and hold them there, exerting a gentle pressure for a moment or two before gently lifting them.

j)   When working with your partner she could lie on her back while you massage her from behind. If she is uncomfortable lying flat then try placing a pile of cushions behind her so that her back and head are well supported.

Massage for pregnancy and labour

Once you have begun with feet, hands, and face you will find that you can continue to explore the whole body intuitively in the same way. With time, patience and a little practice you will begin to discover the magic you have in your hands.

The following ways of massaging are particularly helpful during pregnancy and labour. At all times remember to spend a few minutes breathing deeply with your partner and then stay in tune with her breathing rhythm as you massage.

BACK AND SHOULDER MASSAGE

Your partner should sit in a comfortable resting position with knees apart, either on the floor, leaning forward on to a pile of cushions or else facing backwards on a chair, leaning on its back rest. Place yourself comfortably behind her so that you are well positioned to massage her back.

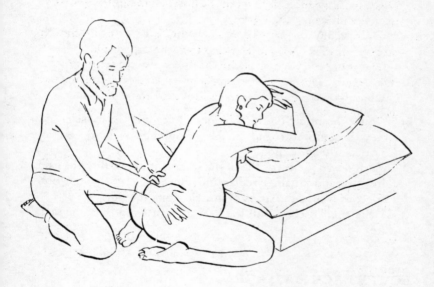

a) Start by using the flat of your hands and firmly and gently stroke down the spine from the neck to the tailbone using one hand after the other in quick succession. This kind of massage is very calming and helps to relieve shiveriness in labour.

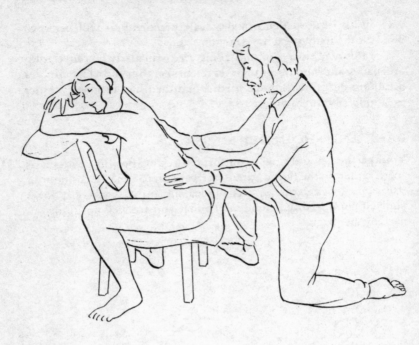

b) Now concentrate on the shoulders, kneading the muscles until they become soft and pliable, stopping to work on any particularly tense spots.
c) Work down the vertebrae of the spine with your thumbs using pressure and small, circular movements. Massage the bony ridges as well as the strips of muscle along the sides.
d) Make small arches with the heel of your hand over the sacral area.

LOWER BACK MASSAGE

The lower back bears a lot of extra strain during pregnancy. It is very relieving for your partner to be massaged regularly over the whole sacral area both during the months of pregnancy and especially during labour. Many women experience backache during contractions and massage can make a great difference to their ability to cope with pain.

a) Using the flat of your hand try making smooth, circular movements over the skin of the whole lower back. During labour when you may do this for several hours it is advisable to use some talcum powder to prevent irritation of the skin. Try doing this massage with your partner in the all–fours position. Ask her to rotate her hips and breathe deeply as if in mid-contraction and tune in to her movements and breathing as you work.

b) Try the same thing again only this time use both hands and work from the spine outwards, over the buttocks and down the thighs. Then repeat the movement, starting again at the spine.

c) Try a deeper pressure massage over the bones of the lower back and sacrum, using your thumbs to dissolve tension and pain.

d) Place your palm over the very end of the spine and use the heel of your hand to exert a gentle pressure upwards against the tailbone or coccyx. Many women find this movement very helpful in labour.

ABDOMINAL MASSAGE

During pregnancy it is very pleasant for both mother and baby to have the abdomen gently massaged. Use a good vegetable oil and the flat of your hand to make smooth, circular movements.

In labour many women enjoy having the lower part of their belly massaged during contractions. When the contractions are very intense, however, most women prefer a very light and gentle touch over this area. Try using just the very tips of your fingers and stroking rhythmically across the lower belly.

PERINEAL MASSAGE

Many midwives recommend massage of the soft tissues of the pelvic floor in preparation for birth. Your partner may prefer to do this herself but it is easier when done by another. A good olive oil should be used and gently massaged into the whole area, while you stretch the perineal muscles with your fingers from side to side. In many parts of the world where birth is not medically aided this is done for several weeks before a birth. Preparing the perineal tissues in this way helps to make the muscles more elastic and supple and to prevent unnecessary tearing at birth.

It is also very helpful to do deep-pressure massage over the pelvic bones and in the groin as this will help your partner to release pain and tension in this area.

5 Labour and birth

Your partner will probably go into labour at some time within the fortnight before or after her expected due date. The length of a normal pregnancy varies and in fact many women start labour after the estimated date.

When the baby is ready to be born, hormones secreted by the mother's pituitary gland trigger off the muscular action of her uterus which begins to contract rhythmically at periodic intervals. These contractions gradually draw up the cervix so that it thins out and then slowly opens until it is wide enough for the baby's head to pass through. Once the cervix is open the uterus contracts from above and pushes the baby down the pelvic canal to birth. The whole process takes place automatically, provided the mother is able to relax and allow her body to respond instinctively.

To sum up

★ The early part of labour, when the cervix thins and opens up, is called the *first stage*.

★ The expulsive part, when the baby is pushed through the birth canal and is born, is called the *second stage*.

★ The *third stage* follows immediately after the baby is born and involves the first contact between mother and baby and the separation and expulsion of the placenta and membranes (afterbirth).

Though all births have these three stages in common, the length of labour and the frequency and strength of the contractions varies tremendously. Experientially too, it is difficult to generalize as no two births are quite alike and what may seem long and arduous to one woman may be easy for another.

Starting

Quite often there is a long period of waiting for labour to start, when it seems as if it will never happen, or, alternatively, it can begin unexpectedly early. In the last few days of pregnancy many women experience a pre-labour – a few hours of mild contractions here and there, which are in fact the very early beginnings but not labour proper. On the other hand some women go straight into labour.

There are, however, some common signs that labour is imminent and your partner could experience any of the following signs:

★   The baby has periods of quietness and moves less than usual.
★   The membranes could break, causing the amniotic fluid to gush out or leak out slowly. This can happen a day or a few hours before or else during labour. Sometimes the membranes remain intact until the baby is actually born.
★   An unusual dull ache in the lower back.
★   An ache rather like a period pain in the lower belly.
★   A feeling of shiveriness that is uncontrollable. This often happens just before or at any stage during the labour and is the body's way of releasing tension. Deep breathing and a calming massage can be helpful.
★   Diarrhoea or frequent emptying of the bowels. This is nature's way of clearing the body in readiness for birth.
★   The plug of mucus which seals the cervix during pregnancy may be discharged. This is known as a 'show'. The mucous usually contains a little blood which can be bright red or a pinky brown colour.
★   Regular contractions.

It is wise in the days before birth for both of you to make sure you get enough rest and sleep. Labour can start at any time of the day or night and can last anything from one hour to thirty-six. A first labour is usually longer than that of subsequent births. The average length of a first birth is eight to sixteen hours, but a duration of around twenty-four hours is not uncommon.

EATING IN LABOUR

The body has a natural tendency to empty before birth in order to make way for the baby. A woman in labour is unlikely to be comfortable with a large or indigestible meal in her stomach. Some women experience quite a bit of nausea in labour and from time to time the stomach can be taken over by an expulsive reflex. After this passes the woman usually feels relieved and relaxed and it is an effective way of releasing tension.

Although it is not advisable to eat heavily during labour, it is very important to keep the level of blood sugar stable and also to provide the mother with some source of energy and nourishment. If the blood sugar of a woman in labour runs low, she will turn very pale and suffer a period of very low energy and spirits and the labour will slow down or could even stop. This condition is known as 'ketosis' and can be detected by testing a sample of urine.

It is easy to avoid this problem by ensuring that your partner has a light meal when labour starts. Something like yoghurt, a soft boiled egg, toast and honey is ideal. If she becomes hungry in labour, a very liquid but nourishing soup is excellent. In fact if the labour is long she should have a few spoonfuls at regular intervals throughout. Chicken or miso soup are ideal. Regular drinks of something sweet – red grape or apple juice, honey in hot water, or a herbal tea such as raspberry leaf or camomile – are helpful. (Avoid citrus juices which are too acidic.)

If your partner does become ketotic two or three glucose tablets and a sweet drink should remedy the situation. In very strong labour regular sips of water will be enough and some 'Rescue Remedy' if she gets tired (see page 93).

Do remember to feed yourself as well! Hospitals often have no provision for hungry partners in the labour ward so bring a picnic with you.

The first stage of labour

This is usually the longest part of the labour and involves the gradual opening of the womb.

WHAT HAPPENS TO THE UTERUS

Before labour starts the cervix is about 1½ inches thick. Hormones cause it to soften and become 'ripe' in readiness for birth. The early contractions work on the lower part of the uterus, drawing up the cervix so that it thins out. This is called 'effacing' and can take place before labour actually starts.

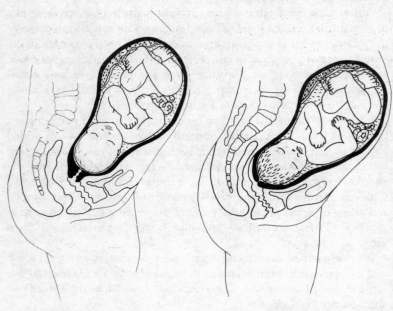

The baby in the womb
before labour starts

The cervix is drawn up and
'thins' in early labour

WHAT HAPPENS TO YOUR PARTNER

Once labour is properly established the contractions come at regular intervals, like waves. Each contraction starts gently, becomes stronger as it reaches a peak and then eases as it wears off.

Every labour has a rhythm of its own and will vary from one woman to another. Some women start off with contractions thirty minutes apart, others with them five or ten minutes apart. They might be quite random at first but will eventually settle into a regular pattern as labour becomes established. As the labour progresses they get more powerful and closer together until eventually, in strong labour, they are three or four minutes apart.

At the peak of the first stage the intervals between contractions last about thirty seconds. Each contraction works to draw the cervix open a little so that it gradually becomes wide enough to allow the baby's head to pass through. This process is known as the dilation of the cervix from 0–10 centimetres.

As the dilation progresses the contractions increase in strength and also get longer. The mild, early contractions last about twenty to thirty seconds. About halfway through the first stage (at about 5 centimetres' dilation) they may be forty-five to fifty seconds long. At the end of the first stage (8–10 centimetres' dilation), when the contractions are at their strongest, they last about a minute to a minute and a half.

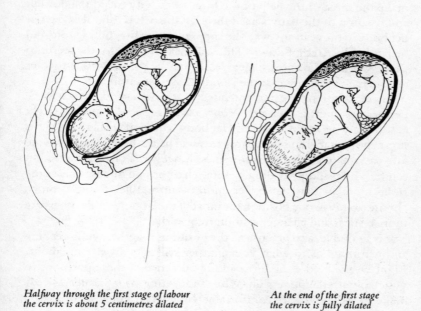

Halfway through the first stage of labour the cervix is about 5 centimetres dilated

At the end of the first stage the cervix is fully dilated

WHAT HAPPENS TO THE BABY

While the cervix is thinning and dilating the baby's head presses down on to it, helping it to open. Pressure from the contracting uterus pushes the baby downwards so that his head gradually passes down lower into the pelvic canal, while the cervix draws up around it. By the time the first stage is over the baby's head has passed more than halfway through the open cervix ready for birth.

The baby's head rotates in a spiral as it passes through the birth canal. Before labour starts, the widest diameter of the baby's head engages in the widest diameter of the pelvic brim, which is from side to side. During labour as it descends it turns so that in the second stage the widest diameter of the head passes through the widest diameter of the mother's pelvis which is from front to back (pubic bone to coccyx).

Positions and movements for the first stage

By using upright positions during the first stage your partner can make the most of the help of the force of gravity to aid the descent and rotation of the baby's head through the pelvis. She also can use her body to move in any way she chooses to ease the contractions and help the baby to come down. This will make it easier for the uterus to do its work without resistance, lessening the pain for your partner and helping to ensure that the labour progresses well.

These positions are not intended as a series of exercises to be performed during labour. Your partner should move freely according to her own instincts. Her body will soon tell her how she is most comfortable and invariably this will be the best position for the safe passage of the baby. Sometimes, however, a tactful suggestion can be a help and providing a stool, chair or pile of cushions at the right moment can make her more comfortable. Some women choose to stay in one position for most of the labour, while others are more restless and change position frequently.

It is a good idea to practise all the positions together while keeping an open mind as to what your partner will actually use in labour. Eight weeks before the birth add the practice of these positions to your daily stretching session. While supporting your partner, always make sure that you are comfortable yourself. If you are not at ease then your discomfort will affect her. Combine the positions explained below with deep breathing and massage and work together until you are completely familiar with the movements and can discover and invent your own variations.

STANDING AND WALKING

When the contractions become strong enough in the first stage many women like to start by standing or walking, leaning forward during the contractions. This will promote a shorter labour, better circulation and is less tiring and painful than lying down. Your partner may like to be held during contractions or to lean forward on to a wall. Some women enjoy very close body contact with their partners and others prefer to support themselves independently. Your partner may like to walk slowly or fast and could easily invent her own 'birth dance'. Rotating her hips in circles or rocking during contractions can ease and sometimes remove the pain. Indeed in ancient Greece pregnant women were taught a dance in preparation for birth. Belly dancing was originally invented and used for childbirth. Many couples enjoy practising to music.

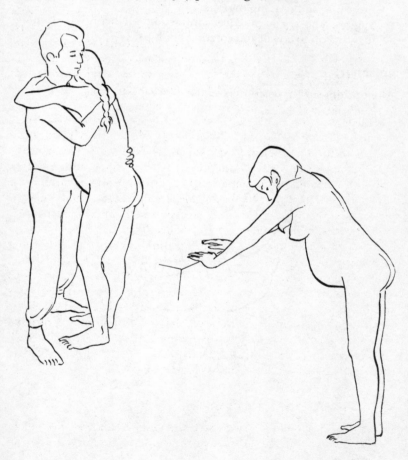

Practise with your partner

* Stand with your feet apart. Rotate your hips, making a circular movement. At the same time breathe deeply, in through the nose and out through the mouth and imagine that you are breathing through a contraction in labour.
* While your partner continues like this, you try standing beside her, breathing with her and massaging her lower back in circles with the palm of your hand. Tune into her rhythm so your massage harmonizes with her movements.
* Try holding her in your arms, her whole body leaning against yours, her head on your shoulder. Massage her back while breathing and moving together.
* Suggest she try a practice contraction on her own, leaning forward on to a wall and rotating her hips.

SITTING

Any upright sitting position is suitable for labour.

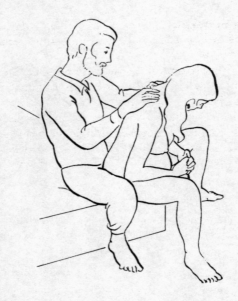

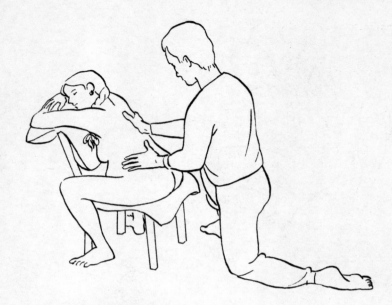

Practise with your partner

* Sit on the floor, back to back and tune into each other's breathing.
* Have your partner sitting on a low stool or chair with her legs wide apart and trunk leaning forward. You could try massaging her back as she breathes through a contraction.
* Have your partner sitting astride a chair facing backwards with her head resting on the back of the chair or a pillow. Kneel behind her and tune into her breathing rhythm while massaging her back.

SQUATTING

Squatting is the ideal position for labour. It opens the pelvis to its widest and intensifies the contractions. Your partner may like to squat either during or in between contractions.

Practise with your partner

* Your partner should squat on a low stool or pile of books, knees as wide apart as possible and body leaning forward. Breathe deeply together for a minute or so, imagining that she is breathing through a contraction.

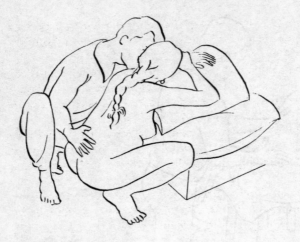

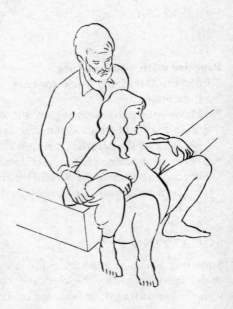

* This time try squatting in between the contractions. Your partner should stand up and breath through a contraction, then return to a squatting position once the contraction is over.
* Next time your partner takes a bath, suggest that she tries

squatting sideways in the water, leaning forward on to the side of the bath. You could use a sponge to bathe her back and shoulders with warm water.

* Both squat on your toes, then come forward to kneel on your hands and knees, then come back to squatting. Practising moving from squatting to kneeling and back will help to make it easy to change positions instinctively in labour.

* Place a large pile of cushions in front of your partner. Help her to squat so that she can lean forward, resting her head on the cushions. Place a small, firm cushion under her heels for extra comfort.

* Sit on a chair with your partner squatting between your knees. She could either face you or rest her back against your body, supporting herself by leaning on your thighs.

KNEELING

Most women instinctively kneel forward as the contractions become very intense. This is a very useful position for the late first stage for a very fast labour, or if the baby is lying in the posterior position. It helps to reduce pain, especially backache, and helps the baby to rotate inside the pelvic canal.

Use a cushion during labour to protect your partner's knees.

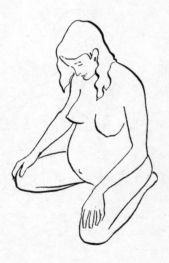

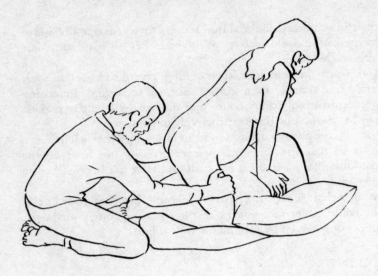

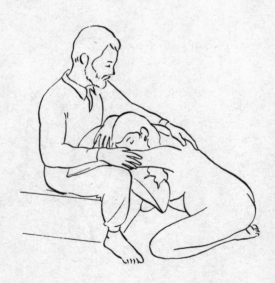

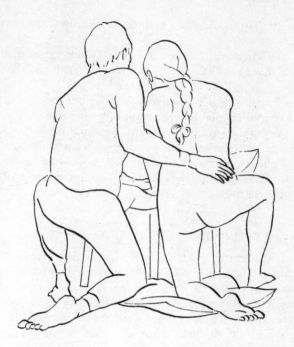

Practise with your partner

* Kneel on all-fours. Slowly rotate your hips, making a circular movement, and at the same time concentrate on the rhythm of your breathing. Breathe in through your nose and out through your mouth. Pay special attention to the exhalation, as if breathing through a contraction in labour.
* While your partner continues in this way, kneel beside her and massage her lower back.
* Try the same thing with your partner kneeling with her trunk upright.
* Try the same thing with your partner kneeling forward on to a pile of cushions so that her body is supported in a resting position.
* Sit on a chair while your partner kneels forward on to your lap.
* Try a kneeling position in the bath, making the water as deep as

possible. You could use a sponge to rinse her back with warm water.

* Try half kneeling on one knee only, while bending the other knee. Change to the other leg for the next contraction.

Note

Any kneeling position is suitable for labour but the amount of help from gravity will depend on the angle of your partner's trunk. If she is more upright then gravity will help more, so kneeling upright will intensify the contractions and kneeling in a forward position will moderate them. If labour is slow she should use more upright positions. If it is fast then the lower kneeling positions will be more comfortable for her.

COPING WITH PAIN

Labour pains are usually felt across the lower abdomen, in the lower back or inner thighs. The pain of childbirth differs from the pain of injury, or from a headache or toothache. Although at times it can be extremely intense, it is a positive pain which brings birth to a child. There are some women who experience completely painless childbirth and many for whom the pain is only a secondary consideration. For the majority of women, however, the stronger contractions are certainly painful and will take them to the limit and possibly beyond the limit of what they can cope with.

Fear, tension and expectation will increase pain as will an environment where there is insensitivity to what the mother is experiencing. If her attendants are unconfident about her ability to cope, the pain will be worse. If she is expected to lie down, the pain will increase as her body will have to fight against gravity rather than be helped by it.

Most women giving birth actively can manage to cope with the inevitable pain if they have the right support and encouragement. Very few women who are free to use their bodies as they choose ever think about using artificial means of pain relief. However, on the other hand, if your partner finds the pain unbearable and decides to make use of pain-reducing methods, it is important to support her in her choice.

The pain of labour is not continuous but is felt mainly at the peak of each contraction. Between contractions it usually melts away and your partner may feel an equivalent pleasure in the release which for some can be quite ecstatic. Essentially it is a matter of taking each contraction as it comes, getting over the top of it, then resting before the next one.

How you can help

★ Have faith in your partner's ability to cope. She may need to be left alone to go through these intense feelings.

★ Keep yourself centred and don't let your own anxiety get in the way.

★ Remind yourself and her too, that once she has her baby in her arms she won't even remember these pains that seem so unbearable now.

★ See if you can change the environment to make it easier for your partner to relax and sink more deeply into what she is experiencing. You can do this by dimming the light, suggesting a bath or shower, taking her for a walk, putting on some music that she likes or fixing a fresh pile of cushions.

★ For those who use homoeopathics there are some remedies which are very helpful in labour. You can buy them at a homoeopathic pharmacy and have them at hand in labour. In the early first stage or at the onset of labour use one dose of Arnica 200 in tablet form. Another dose can be given later on if necessary.

In transition use 'Rescue Remedy'. This is best in tincture form. Use ten drops given directly in the mouth or in a little water.

★ Suggest that your partner changes position.

★ Give her a hot-water bottle.

★ Try massaging her if she asks you to.

★ Remember that pain can also be a message that something is amiss. Listen very carefully to what your partner is saying. If she is finding the pain really unbearable, believe her.

Transition: the end of the first stage

WHAT HAPPENS TO THE UTERUS

The end of the first stage, when the uterus is nearing full dilation (8–10 centimetres) is often called the transition stage. It is like a bridge between the first stage, in which the womb opens, and the second, when the baby is actually born. Transition can last anything from a few minutes to two or three hours, and by the end of transition the womb will be fully open and ready to expell the baby.

The contractions can be very long and intense, last between one and one and a half minutes each, with very short intervals in between.

WHAT HAPPENS TO YOUR PARTNER

Transition is sometimes the most difficult part of the labour, with very long and intense contractions, which are usually very painful. But it is generally not a good idea to use any pain relief at this stage because, by the time it takes effect, your partner will probably be ready to give birth to her baby.

She may begin to feel the urge to bear down starting at the same time as the final dilating contractions. This can be very confusing for her and she may feel at a loss for what to do – despairing and exhausted and possibly nauseous. You may also find that she is very irritable at this time. This is very common and midwives usually take it as a sign that the birth is imminent! As the person closest to her, you may find yourself the target of her irritability, but as soon as the second stage starts she will probably have a new rush of energy.

WHAT HAPPENS TO THE BABY

At this time the baby's head descends right down to the base of the pelvis and passes through the cervix as it opens to its widest. The baby's head presses against the lower bowel, which can give the mother very anal sensations similar to the urge to defecate. The baby's head rotates to pass under the pubic bone and his spine starts to arch, ready to pass out of the pelvic outlet in the second stage.

WHAT YOU CAN DO TO HELP

While helping a woman in transition it is important not to disturb her concentration. She is on the brink of giving birth and her state of consciousness is very deep and open at this time. Everything she is experiencing is very intense and she needs to let herself go and sink into herself. You may best be able to help by leaving her to it – or she may want very close support and body contact, and as partner this may be the time when you can be especially useful. Your moral support and encouragement can help her to relax and persevere through this last difficult patch. Remind her that her baby will soon be born and that she has done and is doing very well.

She may need time to surrender and let go to actually give birth to her baby. Most women instinctively adopt the kneeling forward position at this time, but any of the positions suitable for the first stage can be used and during a long transition changing position can be very helpful. It can also help to take a warm bath.

Breathing together, concentrating on the exhalation, giving her frequent sips of water, a cool sponge or face cloth between contractions, a stretch up – lifting her arms over her head – or holding and massaging her are all ways to help if she wants or needs them.

Anterior Lip

This sometimes occurs before full dilation and it means that the front rim or lip of the cervix is still not quite fully taken up. The midwife will probably feel this rim just in front of the baby's head, and though your partner may feel quite a strong urge to bear down she may be asked by the midwife to try not to until this last bit of cervix is dilated.

In this case suggest that she use the knee-chest position, ie. kneeling forward on her hands and knees and placing her head down and bottom up. In this position the contractions are more comfortable and the front rim of the cervix has room to come up. If your partner feels like pushing, suggest that she blow instead, as if blowing out a candle three feet away.

After three or four contractions the anterior lip will probably have gone. It is not advisable to resist the pushing urge for long, as this can have the effect of stopping the contractions.

The second stage of labour

WHAT HAPPENS TO THE UTERUS

Once the cervix reaches full dilation (10 centimetres), the uterus is open and ready to expel the baby. The expulsive contractions come from the top part of the uterus and are quite different from the earlier contractions which worked to draw up and open the cervix. Your partner may feel the powerful contractions of the second stage beginning just before full dilation. They are usually experienced as a feeling of pressure in the lower bowel quite similar to the urge to defecate. On the other hand she may not feel any contractions at all for a while. In some cases the second stage follows immediately after the cervix is fully dilated and sometimes there is a break in which very little happens. This can last anything from a few minutes to half an hour or so and is a good opportunity for your partner to rest or even sleep until the second stage begins.

The second stage is usually much shorter than the first, lasting from a few minutes to two or three hours. The average length of the second stage is thirty to forty minutes. The uterus contracts firmly from above and presses downwards, pushing the baby further down into the pelvic canal. The intervals between contractions are longer than at the end of the first stage and can last between two and five minutes. Your partner can make the most of these breaks to rest before the next contraction.

WHAT HAPPENS TO YOUR PARTNER

The contractions of the second stage are usually very powerful. Many women, however, find this stage very enjoyable. Some find the sensations of actually giving birth orgasmic and they often describe an ecstasy which is one of the most profound experiences of a lifetime. When a couple share the birthing together, the supporting partner as an active participant is deeply involved. For you, too, then these moments can be momentous and extremely emotional and moving.

For some women the second stage takes place very rapidly and easily of its own accord, while others need to work hard in order to get the baby born. Many factors are involved – the size and shape of the mother's pelvis, the size and position of the baby's head and the mother's feelings about opening her body and allowing the baby to

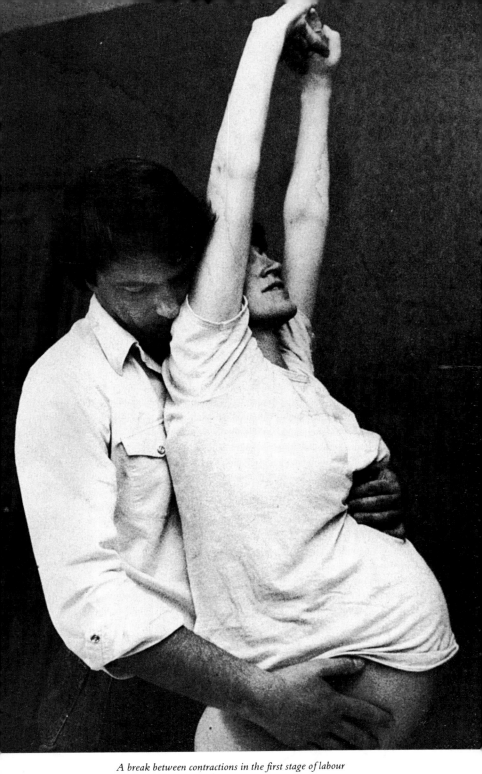

A break between contractions in the first stage of labour

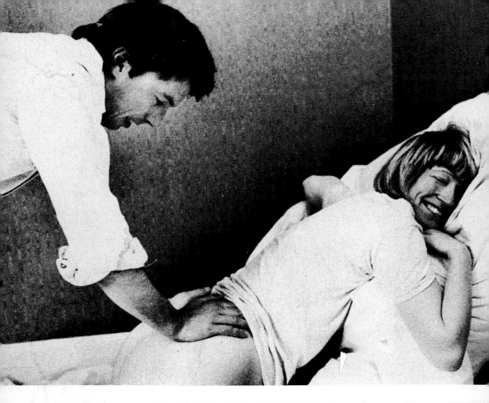

Francis massages Sarah's back in the kneeling position

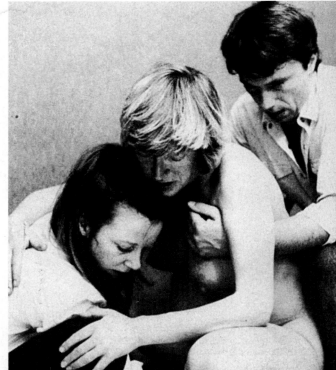

Midwife, Hazel Smith, and Francis support Sarah in the squatting position through strong contractions in the late first stage

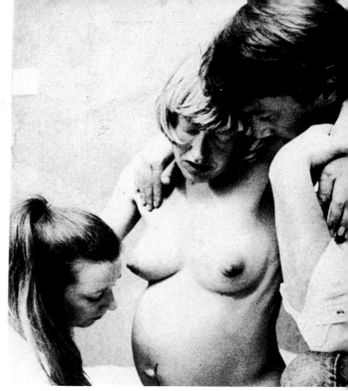

Hazel checks the dilation to see if Sarah is ready to give birth

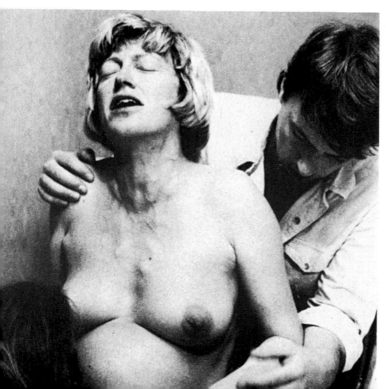

The bearing-down urge begins

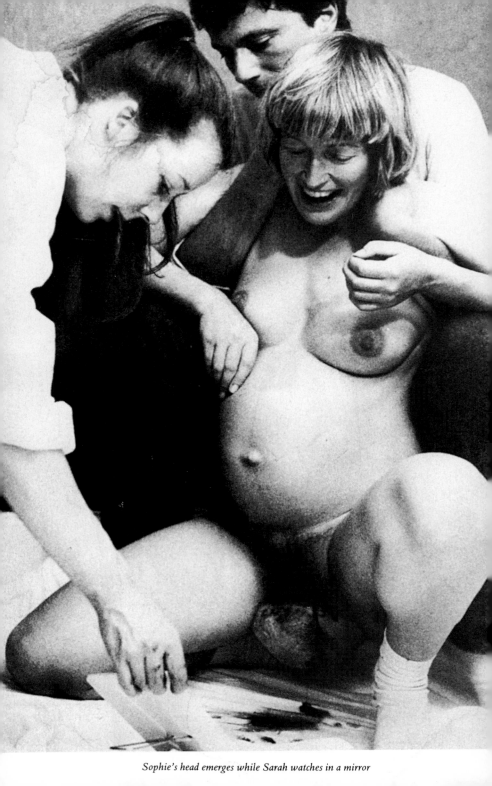

Sophie's head emerges while Sarah watches in a mirror

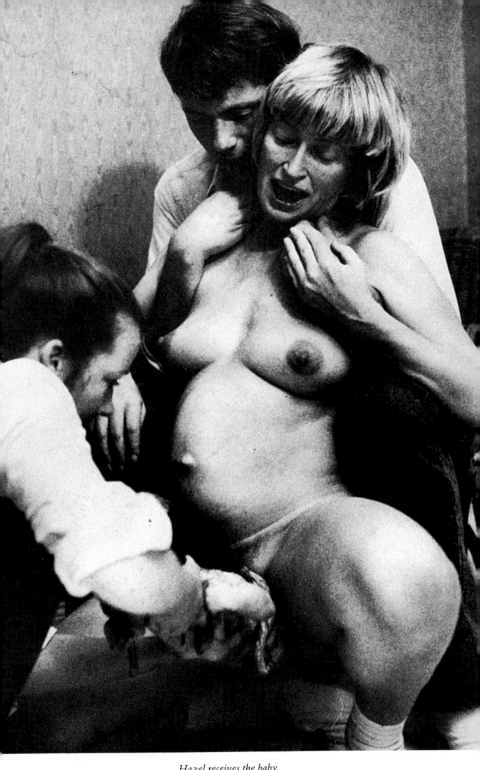

Hazel receives the baby

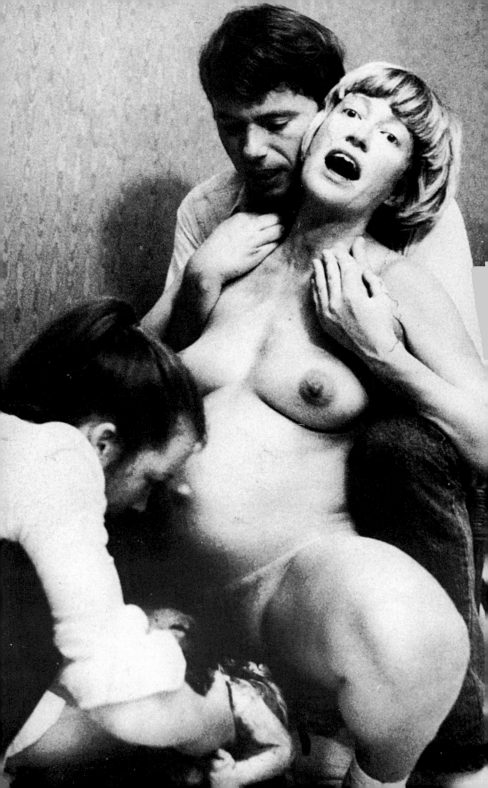

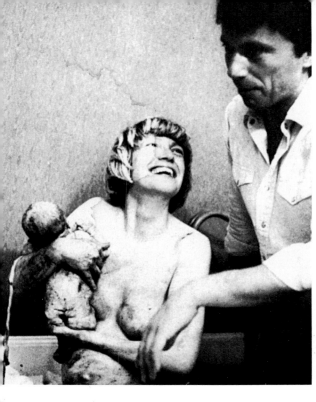

Moments after birth

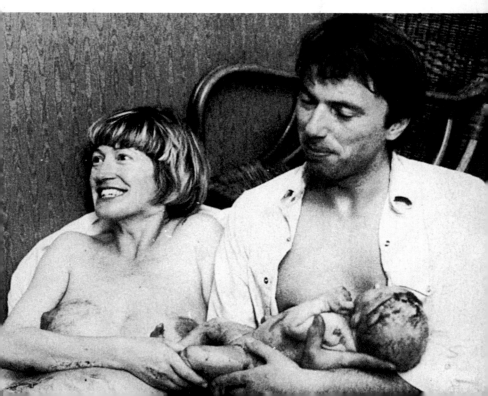

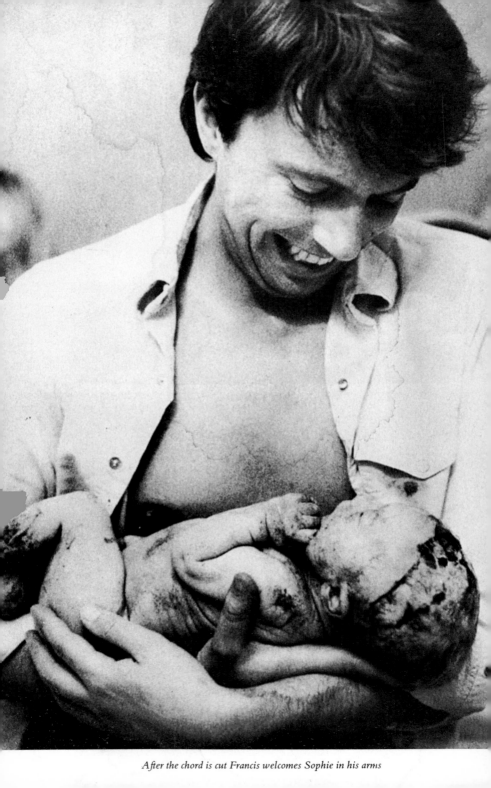

After the chord is cut Francis welcomes Sophie in his arms

be born. Some women are able to do this with ease, while others need time to overcome fear and resistance and to surrender to the powerful process happening inside them. Your partner may well feel at some moments that she is unable to cope, but given time, reassurance and help to relax and surrender, her natural instincts will bring her baby to birth.

Usually after the first stage is over a new wave of energy arises with the expulsive contractions. At some point your partner will feel ready to start pushing her baby out. Her whole body will probably be taken over by the urge to bear down. You may notice a change in her voice and a 'pushing' tone in the sounds she makes. At this stage it is important that she positions her body in a way in which gravity can help her to make full use of the contractions.

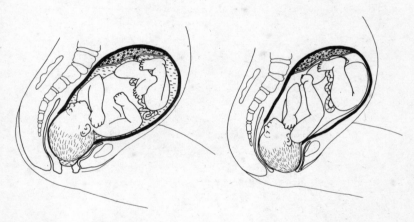

The end of the first stage, transition. The baby's head passes through the cervix in readiness for birth

The early second stage. The baby's head is 'crowning'

WHAT HAPPENS TO THE BABY

In the first part of the second stage the baby's head is pushed right down towards the back of the pelvis (hence the feeling of anal pressure). As the head descends, it rotates slowly and the neck, which was flexed up until this point, begins to extend as it passes through the curved canal of the pelvis, under the pubic bone towards the vagina. As the head reaches the floor of the pelvis, the soft tissues of the vagina begin to bulge and open and the top of the baby's crown begins to show a little more with each contraction. This is called the 'crowning'.

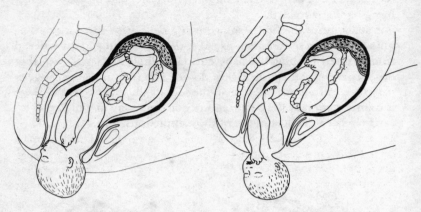

Midway through the second stage the head is out and the baby's body begins to turn

The left shoulder comes out and then the right

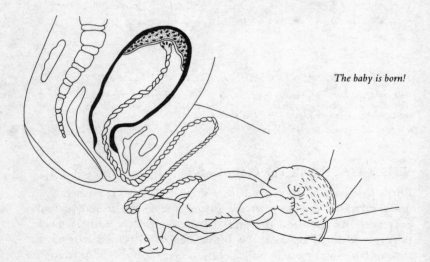

The baby is born!

The soft tissues stretch and yield to the pressure of the descending head which is eventually pushed out. This can happen very fast or gradually in slow stages. Once the baby's head is out the body continues to rotate until the left and then the right shoulder come through and finally the rest of the body.

Immediately after birth the baby will begin to breathe for the first time, will open his eyes and may cry. Depending on the circumstances, some babies are fretful after birth and seem to need to express themselves and to be soothed, while others are born completely tranquil and look about them with a wide-eyed expression of complete innocence that is very moving.

At birth the baby is unlikely to look like the ideal you have been expecting. His skin will probably be quite wrinkled. The head may be a little pointed in shape. This is caused by the skull bones overlapping a little to fit through the birth canal. After a few hours the baby's skin will be smooth and the head will regain its rounded shape.

A newborn baby is often slightly blue or grey in colour immediately after birth, but within minutes, as soon as breathing is established, the colour will change to normal. The skin is covered in a white, creamy substance called vernix. This looks like butter and is highly nutritious. It is absorbed into the baby's skin within hours of the birth. It also acts as a fatty protection against the change of temperature from inside the womb.

Positions and movements for the second stage

There are several positions which are suitable for an active birth. It is a good idea to practise all of them often, starting six weeks before the expected date of birth. In this way you will discover which positions are most comfortable for you both and you will have time to explore ways in which you can adapt to the environment in which the birth is to take place.

If the second stage is very rapid you will probably not have time to change positions, but if it is slow, experiment with different positions until your partner finds the most helpful and comfortable one for her.

SUPPORTING AND BEING SUPPORTED

When two or three people work as a team in order to help a baby to birth it is important that all of you are completely at ease. If one person is uncomfortable tension will be transmitted to the mother and inhibit her progress. For this reason you should practise beforehand.

When supporting make sure you are relaxed and encourage your partner to allow herself to be supported – to let go of her body and give herself to her supporter completely. In this way she will be easier to hold and will be able to surrender to the forces at work inside her.

THE ALL-FOURS POSITION

This position is particularly suitable for a rapid second stage as your partner has more control over the contractions which can sometimes be fast and furious. Many women find this a very comfortable way to give birth.

Your partner should simply position herself comfortably, using a beanbag or pile of cushions to support her body, adjusting the height according to her progress. Alternatively, she could kneel on a firm bed or on the floor. Make sure her knees are protected. If her trunk is upright, gravity will help to bring the baby down. If her head is down and her body more horizontal the contractions will slow down a little and be more moderate. This position may also be helpful if the baby is lying in a posterior position or if the baby has large shoulders, as it encourages the rotation. It is also a good position to use if the birth happens unexpectedly and you need to deliver the baby yourself (see page 139).

It is possible to do internal examinations and even an episiotomy in this position. Turning over into the semi–reclining position for these purposes can involve your partner in a sudden increase in pain.

Practise with your partner
* Practise the kneeling position together and try moving from kneeling on all–fours to half kneeling, half squatting, to sitting upright or to squatting so that this range of movement will come naturally at the time of birth.

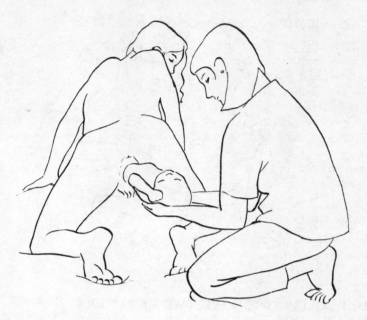

FULL SQUATTING

This position is physiologically ideal for the safe passage of the baby through the birth canal. With the pelvis at its widest, the soft tissues of the pelvic floor are relaxed and the angle of descent is perfect to assist the rotation of the baby's body. The force of gravity helps the work of the uterus.

Practise with your partner

* Sit on a chair with your knees apart and back straight. Ask your partner to squat between your legs, leaning her body against yours and supporting herself on your thighs. Practise standing up, then squatting down again. After the baby is born the mother can simply sit with her legs apart and hold her baby. (See photograph section.)

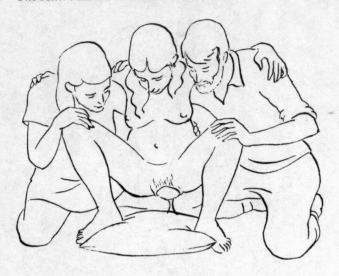

FULL SQUATTING WITH TWO PARTNERS SUPPORTING

The mother should squat down on the floor. Both partners then kneel beside her, coming very close to her and placing one knee each underneath her buttocks and one arm each around her back. She can then squat supported, placing her arms around her supporters' shoulders.

Practise with your partner

★   Try moving from this position to all-fours and back and to standing up and back as these movements may be useful as resting positions during the birth.

★   Although it is best on the floor, if necessary this position can be adapted to a hospital delivery bed if both partners stand on either side of the bed and the mother squats on the bed with her arms around their shoulders and possibly a cushion rolled up under her heels for support. It is a good idea to practise on the kitchen table if you will be giving birth on a hospital bed.

★   Try coming forward on to all-fours or upright kneeling to use as resting positions.

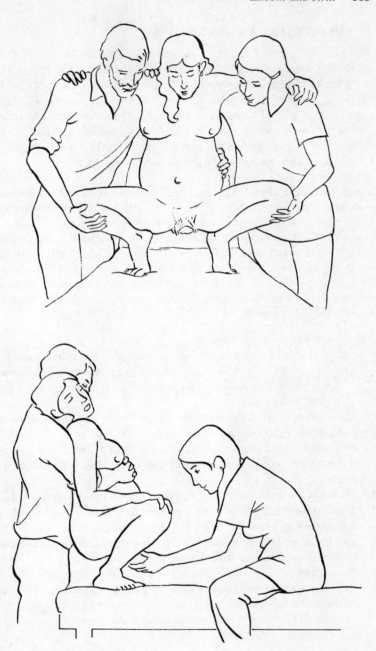

SUPPORTED STANDING SQUAT

This position is physiologically very advantageous as the work of the uterus has maximal help from the downward force of gravity. The baby usually descends more rapidly as a result so this position is particularly useful if the second stage is slow or difficult or if there is any reason to get the baby born as quickly as possible. Many women find this position the easiest. It takes quite a bit of practise for the supporting partner but once you can do it correctly it is easy even for a small partner to support a large woman giving birth.

Try this

Stand with your feet 2 feet apart and pointing forwards. It helps if you have bare feet so that you can grip with your toes. Bend your knees slightly, tighten your buttocks and lean backwards a little.

If you maintain this position and carry the weight of your partner against your pelvis you will be able to support her firmly without strain. If, however, you straighten your knees and bend from your back, you are likely to injure yourself and it may take you longer to recover the full use of your spine than it will take your partner to recover from the birth!

Practise with your partner

★ Stand ready to support her, with your feet apart and straight, knees bent, and buttocks tight, your trunk leaning slightly back. Your partner should stand in front of you, leaning her back against your body.

★ Place your arms under her armpits and give her your hands to hold on to as she squats down. Stand firm and keep your hands relaxed, buttocks tight and carry her weight against your pelvis. Remind her to let go completely and to rest her head and body against you.

★ Hold for a minute or so and then ask your partner to stand up.

★ You do not need to hold your partner in this way until the final contractions, when the baby is about to be born. Up until then and between contractions, she can move as she chooses and can be held in your arms during contractions.

★ Your partner could also give birth facing the other way round with her arms around your neck, the baby being received by the midwife from behind. With the supported standing squat, the firm upward support counterbalances the powerful downward force of the contractions.

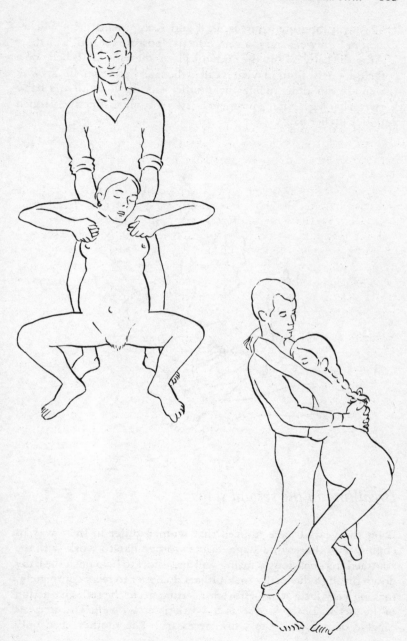

This way of supporting is used and recommended by Michel Odent in Pithiviers and is a very effective posture for active birth.

After the baby is born the midwife places the baby on its belly on a soft cloth on the floor in what is called the safety position. In this way the fluids can drain while the mother sits down with the baby between her legs. After a moment or two she will instinctively touch and pick up her baby.

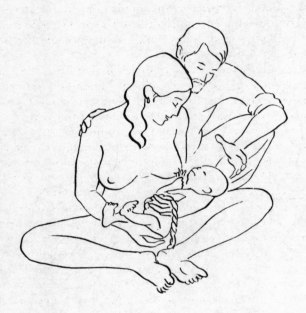

Breathing in the second stage

Over the years I have noticed that women differ in their way of coping with the second stage. Some women like to work with the contractions consciously, using will and effort to help push the baby down through the birth canal. Others do better to relax completely, making very little actual effort and letting go to the reflexive action of the uterus. Both ways seem to work perfectly well. The uterus is capable of doing all the work necessary. The mother need only follow the internal messages from her body to discover her deepest instincts and give birth to her child.

Most birth attendants have been trained to instruct the mother to hold her breath and push vigorously. This approach to the second stage went hand in hand with the reclining posture, when the mother had to work hard against resistance to the force of gravity in order to push her baby out uphill. Research has shown, however, that this kind of strenuous effort seriously reduces the amount of oxygen in the mother's blood and therefore the supply going to the uterus and the baby. This is the stage at which the baby is considered to be most at risk and as good a supply of oxygen as possible is vital to his health and wellbeing.

Another disadvantage of this approach is that often the people assisting the mother are so energetic in their attempts to encourage her and in their instructions to 'push', that she loses contact with her own instinctive messages. This final stage of the birth is a time when everyone present is very excited and often a little anxious too. It is important for everyone to control these feelings, to be calm, outwardly at least, and to give the mother enough time and space to concentrate deeply and to discover her own way of giving birth. She will need encouragement without too much instruction.

The second stage has a rhythm of its own. The contractions come like tidal waves, each giving new force and energy to bring the baby further through the birth canal. The mother will need to find a way of surrendering to this great rhythm within her body and working along with it to get her baby born. It usually takes a few contractions before she can adjust to these new and very powerful sensations.

It is advisable to practise both how to work with the contractions and how to let go and let the uterus do all the work, so that both ways will be available when the time comes. Your partner could practise the following exercises alone or you can join her if you like as it will help you to assist her during the birth.

AWARENESS OF THE PELVIC FLOOR

The muscles of the pelvic floor lie like a hammock across the bottom of the pelvis. They surround the vagina, urethra and anus and the baby has to pass through them to be born. Unlike the uterus, which works automatically, the pelvic-floor muscles are within our conscious control. We can tighten and release them at will. In the final stages of birth they and the surrounding tissues soften and open to release the baby.

To practise your partner should try this

* Squat down on her toes, leaning forwards on to her hands for support, close her eyes and direct her awareness to her pelvic floor.
* Tighten the muscles, pulling them upwards, hold for a few seconds and then gently and slowly release them. Repeat five times.
* Now she should try breathing deeply at the same time, breathing in as she tightens and out as she releases. Repeat five times.

WORKING WITH THE CONTRACTIONS

Once again your partner should squat down, leaning forwards on to her hands. She should imagine that she is in the midst of a contraction. The bearing-down urge and action is similar to the sort of effort made while defecating, but of course takes place in the vagina. She should then try gently bearing down towards her vagina.

To practise try this

* It is difficult to practise this without the actual contractions, so use your imagination. Your partner should take a deep breath before she starts and then push as she breathes out. It is impossible to do this silently and during the actual birth the mother is likely to make a lot of noise as she pushes. This is perfectly natural and although it may sound frightening to others, it is usually very relieving and helpful for her.
* Several small pushes are as effective as one big one.

LETTING GO TO THE CONTRACTIONS

Try this in a comfortable, supported squatting position. Help your partner to relax her whole body, to let go of her head and neck and to allow herself to be completely supported against you.

To practise try this

* Suggest to your partner that she squat down on her toes, close her eyes and direct her awareness to her pelvic floor. Then to imagine that the baby is inside her, his head about the size of a

grapefruit, well down inside the pelvis, ready to be born.
* Remind her to breathe deeply. Each time she breathes out, she should release the pelvic floor, imagining that she is 'breathing' her baby out with each exhalation. While she does so she should direct her attention downward and allow the whole pelvic floor to open and let go while she breathes out.

GIVING BIRTH

At the moment of actually giving birth the baby's head emerges through the vaginal opening. The tissues of the vagina stretch amazingly to allow the head to pass through. For everyone present this is a dramatic moment. The mother is engulfed by a tremendous rush of feelings and sensations within her body.

At this point some women are incapable of any self control and simply surrender to what is taking place within them. Usually just as the baby emerges the mother will cry out – a primal cry which is universal amongst women of all cultures. Some women, however, prefer to work with the midwife and to follow her instructions, panting gently over the peak of each contraction.

To practise your partner should try this
* Squat down on her toes, close her eyes and direct her awareness to her pelvic floor. She should then pant gently, like a dog on a hot day, making the sound 'ha'. Each time she breathes out, she should release the pelvic floor.

The third stage of labour

The third stage begins the moment your partner has her newborn baby in her arms, his naked body against hers. The baby will open his eyes and look up at her face, and yours, as he enjoys the wonder of seeing the world for the first time. The cooler air of the room on the baby's skin will stimulate the breathing response and within a few moments he will be breathing into his lungs. At the same time, while learning to breathe independently, the baby will still be receiving blood from the umbilical cord and placenta.

The rush of emotions felt by the mother, the skin to skin and mouth to nipple contact between her and her baby, all help to stimulate the release of hormones which cause the uterus to contract strongly in order to expel the placenta. This usually takes place within half an hour of the birth but can take longer. This first half hour after birth is an important time for mother, father and baby when they are greeting each other for the first time, and there is no need to rush or stimulate delivery of the placenta.

If the birth has taken place spontaneously in a squatting or kneeling position conditions are optimal for a successful third stage. It is important for the mother to sit really upright as this facilitates the separation of the placenta and is comfortable for perfect contact between mother and baby.

To practise try this
* Ask your partner to sit on the floor with her legs apart as if she has just given birth.
* Stand behind her, with bare feet, so that your legs provide her with support for her back.

At some time during the first half hour the baby will probably start suckling at the breast. This will stimulate the uterus to contract strongly. When your partner feels the contractions coming on to deliver the placenta she should squat or stand up. There is no need for anyone to pull on the cord as she does so (cord traction). This is a dangerous practice. The placenta will come out of its own accord and your partner will enjoy pushing it out as it is smaller and softer than the baby.

6 The environment for birth

I once had the good fortune, as many people do, to witness our cat having her first litter of kittens. When her time to give birth was close she began to investigate the whole house. Finally, when her contractions started she came to call me and ran to the corner of my bedroom, indicating that my wardrobe was the chosen spot. I placed a cardboard box, lined with newspaper, in the dark corner where she was pacing in circles. She allowed my two young children and I to watch her labouring and finally giving birth to five little kittens. It was a marvellous lesson in instinct. She knew exactly what to do. Apart from one contraction before the birth of the first kitten, when she cried out in what seemed to be pain, she purred loudly through the whole experience, licking each kitten before the next one was born.

A woman choosing her attendants and place of birth, like our cat, needs to explore all the possible alternatives and then arrive at her decision in the place she feels most comfortable. As her partner you can help her to investigate the field and see what is open to her, you can discuss the relevant issues and your own preferences but ultimately the choice should be hers. For a woman, choosing the place to have her baby is a nesting *instinct* and the best thing you can do is to support her in her search and trust her feelings and inclinations in making her choice.

Today many women are cut off from the built-in knowledge of birthing which is natural and instinctive amongst animals and primitive peoples. A woman having her first baby is unlikely to have witnessed birth at first hand. She probably does not regard birth as a normal physiological event and a commonplace occurrence. Unwittingly, through fear, ignorance and insecurity she may well choose a place to have her baby which later she could easily regret. Thousands of women, no longer trusting their instincts, passively accept the nearest hospital as the most convenient place to have their babies, and without much thought or enquiry automatically step into an institution where they become 'patients' and the whole affair is taken out of their hands.

Choosing the right environment and attendants whom one trusts, is a prerequisite for a successful outcome. Every woman can and should approach birth with awareness, confident in her own birthing instinct and feeling comfortable and secure in her choice of the place of birth and attendants. As her partner it is important that when helping her to discover what is best for her you should have a basic knowledge and understanding of the choices available.

An active birth can take place in any environment where the attitudes of the attendants and the atmosphere are right. It can be within a hospital suite or in the simplest and most basic room at home. No expensive equipment is necessary. A beanbag or a pile of comfortable cushions, a low stool for squatting and perhaps a chair are all that are needed. What is essential is that you should both feel comfortable and at home, so that your partner can get on with the task of giving birth undisturbed. She should be supported lovingly by all those present in the room and encouraged to trust her instincts. Their attitude of mind is vital to her comfort. So too is her freedom. She should be able to let herself go, be completely uninhibited and use her body as she wishes, with her privacy, authority and dignity respected by all those attending her.

Our cat demonstrated very clearly the most important considerations in choosing her place of birth. She picked a dark corner in one of the quietest spots in the house where she was least likely to be disturbed or interfered with.

Professor Cornelius Naaktgeboren, a Dutch zoologist famous for his studies of animals giving birth, has demonstrated how fear and interruption at this time create tension which actually slows down and stops the progress of labour. The secretion of hormones in a woman's body, which trigger off and stimulate her contractions, are inextricably connected with her emotions. If she is unduly afraid or uncomfortable, the progress of her labour will be adversely affected. Sometimes the mere presence of a person in the room with whom she does not feel at ease can inhibit her contractions, let alone a whole group of students staring at her perineum. If she is tense, stressed and frightened her uterus will tighten and resist its natural tendency to release and open, causing her more pain and more fear, until at last one thing leads to another and she needs help and intervention to give birth to her baby. When birth is uncomplicated, as in over 90 per cent of cases, the safest place for a mother giving birth is one in which she is undisturbed both psychologically and physically.

The attitude of mind of those around her is as vitally important to her comfort, security and wellbeing and the safety of her baby as is her freedom to use her body. It is only under these conditions that a truly instinctive and active birth can take place.

Birth in hospital

In the majority of hospitals a series of obstetric means of managing labour and birth are used routinely. These techniques intervene in the natural course of events and are known as 'the active management of labour'. Many people today suffer under the illusion that hospital is necessarily the safest place to have a baby. Suzanne Arms, in her book *Immaculate Deception* describes what she calls the 'obstetric mentality'. She is writing about typical hospital birth in America where obstetric technology is routinely used to an extreme, but what she says is relevant enough in Britain and many other countries.

> The unspoken assumption of obstetrics today is that what is predictable is certainly more safe than what is not, and the process of birth is not predictable enough. In an effort to control birth and make it predictable, obstetrical science has devised a routine series of interferences designed to 'improve' upon the normal birth. The obstetrician thus patterns his practice in normal birth after his practice in abnormal birth, forcing the majority of women to undergo procedures that are unnecessary for all but a few women. This makes the birth process a more predictable operation for the doctor, even though any interference can create a greater risk to the woman than the original problem it was intended to solve. Whether interferences are worth this risk is a question the physician feels only he is qualified to judge. In her reliance upon

her doctor's authority, the pregnant woman is seldom aware that such decisions are being made over her prone body, and she is rarely informed of the potential dangers to herself and her baby of each and every alteration to the natural process.

Undeniably the wide availability of obstetric help is a godsend to the small number of women and babies at risk in childbirth. However, the widespread and routine use of such intervention calls for a thorough and careful investigation when choosing the place of birth.

Most hospitals invite expectant couples to come on a tour of the labour ward at some time in the latter part of the pregnancy. In some hospitals ante-natal classes and fathers' evenings are available but these too are usually held at the end of the pregnancy. During the months of pregnancy the crowded and busy ante-natal clinics rarely afford the woman or her partner time to ask questions or to find out much about hospital policy. All too often it happens that the couple only begin to find out about this when it is too late to find an alternative.

It is both sensible and perfectly within a woman's right to make her enquiries and to visit the hospital before deciding to book in for the birth. You can encourage and assist her to do so by suggesting you both make an appointment to talk to the senior midwife or relevant consultant and accompany her if she wishes. This will help the hospital to know more about how your partner would like the birth to be and will make it easier for them to accommodate you both. If the consultant attaches a letter to your partner's notes, stating that she is intending to give birth actively, this will help the staff to assist you when you come in during labour.

Before visiting the hospital it will be helpful for you both to have some understanding and knowledge about the obstetric techniques that are generally used so that you can consider the pros and cons involved. This basic knowledge will be useful to you both in your role as partner and will also later on, if and when the need for intervention arises in labour. Try to accompany your partner on a tour of a labour ward, early on in the pregnancy if possible, and ask in as much detail as you both want to what interventions are used, whether they are performed as a matter of routine or whether one is free to refuse them.

ADMISSION PROCEDURES

These vary in different hospitals but generally upon arrival there are some forms to fill in and then the mother is taken by a midwife to an 'admission room' where she is 'prepared' for labour. Her blood pressure and the baby's position and heartbeat are checked. The she is examined internally to check how far her cervix has dilated. In some hospitals the membranes are routinely ruptured at this point, sometimes without the mother's consent or knowledge.

In some hospitals the pubic hair is shaved or trimmed. This practice is completely unnecessary and humiliating to the woman in labour and has no medical advantage. In fact the prickly new hairs growing after the birth are more likely to *cause* an infection.

Another part of the routine is to give the mother an enema or suppository to empty her bowels. It is not necessary to do so, though it may be helpful if the mother is constipated. In most cases, however, the bowels tend to empty naturally just before labour anyway. Some women are quite happy to have an enema and feel more comfortable afterwards but many find this extremely intrusive and it can be very uncomfortable indeed causing severe cramps, nausea and vomiting if done in strong labour. The important thing is that the mother should have the freedom to refuse if she wishes to.

After the enema a shower or bath is offered. This can be a good opportunity for the mother to relax and she should be encouraged to take her time if she is enjoying it. After the bath she will be given a hospital gown to wear and she is ready to enter the labour ward.

Although the progress of the labour and the wellbeing of mother and baby need to be checked, the way this is done often makes the mother feel that she is a patient and is handing over responsibility to the experts at this stage. The half hour or so that this takes can be a most difficult time for the woman, depending of course on the way she is treated. She is already in labour and has moved from the familiar environment of her home into the unfamiliar surroundings of the hospital. Often her labour will slow down or stop completely until she is able to settle down, relax and find her rhythm again.

In many hospitals partners are asked to leave the room or may have gone to park the car for example. It is a good idea for you to stay together if possible at this time as the mother will be used to your support and may be in particular need of it. You could well be able to help her keep a sense of continuity by remaining at her side and calmly concentrating and breathing through each contraction as usual.

It will be helpful if the mother's notes already have the information that she would like to give birth actively. The checking of the foetal heart and the dilation of the cervix will disturb her less if she is not expected to lie down. She may also prefer to wear a nightdress of her own rather than the hospital gown. In some hospitals partners are expected to wear a sterile hospital gown and sometimes a paper cap and mask. These look ridiculous and are all completely unnecessary as you are unlikely to cause an infection. However, you may feel that it is worth accepting these minor humiliations for the sake of being there and perhaps getting your way on more important issues.

GLUCOSE DRIP

In some hospitals it is recommended that every woman should be connected throughout labour to an intravenous glucose drip in order to keep up the level of glucose in her blood. This goes along with the practice of not allowing a woman in labour to eat. The reason usually given is that she may need a Caesarean section and should therefore have an empty stomach. This is what Suzanne Arms calls the 'just-in-case syndrome'. It means that every birth is regarded as a potential Caesarean section and a woman having a perfectly normal but long labour must then go for hours without food (see page 80). Of course, if the mother is attached to a drip, she is again immobilized and reclining. There is also new evidence that too much sugar in labour may cause postnatal jaundice in babies.

Monitoring

Monitoring means listening to and checking the heartbeat of the baby inside the womb. It is done in pregnancy each time the woman has a check-up and is continued at regular intervals throughout labour until the baby is born. There are many ways to listen to a baby's heart. The simplest is to place one's ear against the mother's lower abdomen in the area where the heart can be heard. When partnering a woman for birth, it is a good idea to learn how to do this as it may well be useful during labour if you can help to 'monitor' the baby. Midwives often use a metal or wooden 'ear trumpet' to listen to the heartbeat and a simple home version of this is the cardboard tube from an empty toilet roll. An ordinary stethoscope can also be used. This is helpful for an active birth as the mother can remain in a comfortable upright position while her attendant can easily get to the lower abdomen.

If you are present at one of the monthly check-ups you could ask the midwife or doctor to show you how to find the heartbeat. A baby's heart beats much faster than an adult's. The heartbeat can be heard from twenty to twenty-four weeks. In early pregnancy you can hear it just over the pubic bones and it can beat as rapidly as 150–60 beats per minute. By full term there should be 120–60 beats per minute. To check the heartbeat, look simultaneously at the second hand of your watch, count the number of beats in 15 seconds and then multiply by 4. For example if you count 32 beats in 15 seconds that makes 128 beats per minute.

ULTRASONIC HEART MONITORS (Doppler or Sonic Aid)

This is a way of listening to the foetal heart by using very mild, high-frequency sound vibrations. The simplest of these machines is a portable version which consists of a small box with a transductor at one end which is held against the mother's abdomen. The heartbeat can then be heard magnified through a little speaker. Domiciliary midwives sometimes carry these. Your GP may well have a slightly larger version in his or her office and hospitals often have them on the labour ward.

These are very useful for a woman wishing to remain active in labour as the transducor, a disc very much like that at the end of a stethoscope, is held on her abdomen and she can continue standing, kneeling or sitting up as she pleases. Although this form of monitoring is not continuous you, as birth partner, can easily learn how to use it and can help by listening regularly to the baby's heartbeat. This is encouraged in one London hospital and indeed it seems logical that being someone who cares deeply about the baby's wellbeing, you will give the best possible care. If the baby is distressed the heartbeat will become irregular or will slow down and this is quite noticeable. This method of monitoring causes no discomfort to the mother. It is also easy for the attendant and as yet there is no evidence to indicate that it can harm the baby, although the long-term effects are untested and some women are reluctant to expose their babies to ultrasound vibrations.

ELECTRONIC HEART MONITORS

These were originally designed for use in the small percentage of problematic births where the baby in the womb is considered to be at risk. In recent years they have become very fashionable and many hospitals insist on their routine use for all women in labour. There are two varieties.

1　The abdominal belt (external monitor)

The mother is expected to lie in a semi-reclining position on the bed and two metal discs, similar to those at the end of a stethoscope, are placed in position on her abdomen. The bottom one records the baby's heartbeat and the top one contains a pressure gauge which records the pressure of the uterus during contractions. These are held in position by two belts which are strapped around the mother's abdomen and are then connected to the monitor, a compact box in a rectangular cabinet at the bedside. The information emerges from this as two continuous printouts resembling brain wave patterns which can be read instantly. The monitor can also amplify the baby's heartbeat. A bleeping light reflects the heartbeat but this can usually be switched off.

2　The scalp electrode (internal monitor)

Here an electrode is attached to the baby's scalp through the cervix which should be dilated at least 1 or 2 centimetres. In order to do this the membranes surrounding the baby must be artificially ruptured (see page 121). The electrode is attached to a catheter which connects it with the monitor. Another catheter, attached to the uterus, will record the pressure of contractions, or an external belt monitor is used. This form of monitoring is supposed to be more accurate than the belt monitor.

Electronic monitoring is useful for high-risk births where intervention is necessary. When birth is induced it is important to monitor the contractions as it can be very dangerous for the baby if they are too strong. For normal labour, however, they cause more problems than they prevent.

The most serious disadvantage is that the monitors confine the mother to the reclining position and immobilize her. In this position her uterus will contract less effectively, the contractions will be more painful and she is more likely to be stressed. Her circulation will slow down as a result of increased pressure on the large blood vessels (the aorta and inferior vena cava), which run along the inside of her spine. Therefore the circulation of blood to and from the uterus will be reduced. As already mentioned this position is the one most likely to *induce* foetal distress, so it seems paradoxical to say the least, to confine the mother to lying back while using a machine to detect the least sign of foetal distress. Artificially rupturing the membranes in order to attach the electrode also significantly increases the risk to the baby.

In addition many women find the belts used for external monitors very uncomfortable. I have tried having an electrode screwed into my hand – it hurts! In fact one obstetrician I know stopped using the scalp electrode routinely after trying it out on his own head. Eighty-five per cent of all babies monitored in this way develop a rash on the spot afterwards, some get an abscess and others are left with a permanent bald spot.

Another disadvantage lies in the fallibility of machines. Electronic monitors break down as often as washing machines. They may also give incorrect information and the way in which the information is interpreted will differ too. Undoubtedly some women are reassured by the use of monitors but for others it has the psychological effect of making them feel that the birth is controlled outside their own body. This is counterproductive to our aim of helping the mother to be in contact with her own internal rhythms and instincts, fully in control of the birth herself.

Electronic monitors have a similar effect on midwives and attendants. The human element is replaced by a machine and the midwife can easily become a machine-minder while the mother in labour is neglected. After a time midwives depending on monitors lose confidence in their own intuition and skills.

TELEMETRIC MONITORING

A recent invention is a form of monitoring using radio waves. This allows the mother mobility and women using it are more comfortable and their labours progress better. However, the drawback is that an electrode still needs to be attached to the baby's scalp and therefore the membranes are ruptured.

In the final analysis the use of electronic monitors seems to be fraught with difficulties. Research shows that the incidence of foetal distress is no less and may even be higher when constant monitoring is used. An experienced attendant checking on the baby's heartbeat and wellbeing is probably a far safer and more pleasant alternative.

Induction

Primitive woman had no 'due date' and indeed the length of a normal pregnancy varies from woman to woman. The due date is only an average estimate and women give birth some time within the two if not three weeks before or after it. These days, however, if labour is late or slow in starting we rarely wait patiently for nature to take its course and different means of inducing the labour are proposed by the birth attendants. The mother is often told, without adequate testing, that if she does not comply the baby will be at risk from postmaturity, the placenta may cease to function adequately or the baby may grow too large. Although sometimes this can be true, all too often it is not and the mother is confronted with a nerve-racking dilemma which she could well do without just before giving birth. What she is very rarely told is how inducing the birth places her baby and herself at considerable risk.

In the 1970s induction was so popular in some hospitals that births were being routinely induced so that all babies could be born in daylight hours or for other purely social reasons. As the dangers of induction are becoming more widely understood this fashion has decreased somewhat, but induced birth is still so common as to demand careful investigation.

Doctors and hospitals have different attitudes to inducing labour. Some like to induce if birth is a few days past the due date, others will wait one week or maybe two. Before choosing the place to have her baby your partner would do well to find out about the hospital policies and statistics on induction. For a small percentage of women induction is an invaluable obstetric help. Good medical reasons for inducing birth may be if the mother has symptoms of pre-eclampsia (see page 135), if she is diabetic or if there is genuine reason to suspect that the placenta is failing and the baby would be safer outside the uterus.

However, a baby born prematurely is at greater risk than one that is slightly overdue and careful tests should be carried out to assess whether there are sufficient medical indications for induction. The placental function can be tested by taking blood and urine samples from the mother to measure the amount of oestrogen which is secreted by the placenta (oestriol tests). The size of the baby can be assessed by an ultrasound scan. If the mother does not have all three of the following symptoms – raised blood pressure, albumin in her urine and oedema (swelling usually on the hands and feet) – and the oestriol test is negative then it is unlikely that an induction is at all necessary merely because labour hasn't started on the due date.

METHODS OF INDUCING BIRTH

Artificial rupture of membranes (ARM, amniotomy)

This is a common way of starting off a labour that is imminent or of accelerating a slow labour.

A sterile, blunt instrument resembling a crochet hook is introduced through the vagina and cervix and the membranes surrounding the baby are torn, causing the amniotic fluid inside to empty. In some hospitals ARM is done routinely as part of the admission procedure.

The membranes, when they are intact, form a barrier which protects the baby inside the uterus from infection. Under normal circumstances the membranes usually break spontaneously towards the end of the first stage of labour. They also cushion and protect the baby's head from the powerful contractions of the uterus which press against it. When the membranes have ruptured there is greater risk of infection to mother and baby and increased pressure, which means that less blood and oxygen goes to the baby's brain. Furthermore, the natural moulding of the skull bones is increased and there is twice as much risk of actual misalignment of the bones. This can cause damage to the baby's brain.

For the mother rupturing the membranes heightens the contractions and it is often difficult for her to cope with this rapid increase in intensity. If an ARM is done before labour is ready to start the procedure may fail and the end result may be a Caesarean section, as many doctors do not feel it safe to wait more than twenty-four hours for the child to be born.

Prostoglandins

These are synthetic versions of the hormone found naturally in semen which has the effect of softening the cervix to allow the sperm to enter the uterus. It usually comes in the form of a pessary which is placed in the vagina or a cream which is applied to the cervix. If labour is imminent prostoglandins may help to start it off. If the birth is not ready to start they probably have no effect and then stronger measures follow.

They are usually applied at night in the hope that labour will have started by the following morning. They have the advantage, when they work, of preventing the need for amniotomy or a drip so that the membranes can remain intact and an active labour can follow.

Oxytocin drip (Syntocinon or Pitocin in the USA)

When pregnancy reaches full term the pituitary gland in the mother produces a hormone called oxytocin which stimulates and regulates the contractions of her uterus throughout labour until after the birth. Obstetric scientists have formulated a synthetic version of this hormone called oxytocin or syntocinon, which they introduce into the mother's bloodstream through an intravenous drip, usually in her arm. She is asked to lie in the semi-reclining position and a catheter is inserted into a vein and then connected to a plastic bag on a stand beside the bed, which contains the hormone solution. This drips at regular intervals into her bloodstream. Usually it begins to take effect almost immediately and as the oxytocin level is much higher than the natural level in the body, the contractions are longer, more powerful and closer together.

Once the labour is chemically induced in this way a heart monitor will probably be used as well and the birth is now medically controlled. If the mother is confined to the semi-reclining position, the same disadvantages to the progress of the labour which have already been described will ensue.

An induced birth is more intense and the pain is usually more difficult to cope with so that the mother is more likely to want analgesics or an epidural. Some women do manage to cope without them though, particularly if they are able to kneel or sit instead of lying down.

When the uterus contracts normally the muscles tighten and during the contraction the baby receives less oxygen as the blood flow is restricted. In the pause between contractions the oxygen level is made up. When birth is induced because intensity and frequency of the contractions is so increased there is more risk of the baby being deprived of oxygen (hypoxia).

The added pressure on the baby's head, particularly if the membranes have been ruptured, heightens the risk of misalignment of the skull bones and compression of the umbilical cord. Research has also shown that the acid–base balance of the mother's and hence the baby's blood is altered by induction and this can be linked with brain damage.

Babies who are born premature as a result of being induced too early are more at risk and more likely to suffer from jaundice. It is important to remember that after the birth the baby is going to have to recover from the effects of the induction. At the time of birth many of the baby's vital organs are only just starting to function and it will be quite a task for the child to cope with these disadvantages as well, particularly if he is born prematurely!

Oxytocin injection (Syntocinon or Ergometrine)

This is an injection given intra-muscularly into the thigh of the mother just as the baby's front shoulder is emerging, often without her consent or knowledge. It is used as a means of inducing the third stage of labour. Most doctors and hospitals insist on continuing this practice, even in places where active birth is otherwise accepted.

Normally, once the baby is born the contact between mother and baby provokes the secretion of natural oxytocin which causes the uterus to contract strongly. This occurs ten to thirty minutes or so after the birth. The new contractions cause the placenta to separate from the wall of the uterus and be expelled.

After an oxytocin injection the placenta separates within minutes. There is then a danger that the uterus will contract strongly and trap the placenta, so attendants like to clamp and cut the umbilical cord and pull the placenta out immediately instead of waiting for the uterus to expel it. This increases the risk of retained placenta and postpartum haemorrhage, although the reason given for its use is that it prevents haemorrhage.

When birth is active, haemorrhage is far less likely. If the mother has given birth spontaneously without intervention there is no reason why her body should not secrete the hormones necessary to separate and deliver the placenta naturally. The squatting position actually facilitates the separation of the placenta in the best possible way. Inducing the third stage completely reverses the normal physiology and can disturb the first contact between mother and baby.

If, on the rare occasion when the mother is bleeding heavily after the birth, the injection can be given at that stage as it only takes thirty seconds to begin to take effect.

ACCELERATION OF LABOUR

If a labour is progressing slowly hospitals are often quick to advise rupturing the membranes as a way of speeding things up or the use of an oxytocin drip. I have found that a lot of patience, a walk, a warm bath or homoeopathic remedies usually work in this situation.

EPISIOTOMY

An episiotomy is a surgical cut about ¾–1 inch long made off to one side of the mother's vagina in order to enlarge the opening. It is usually done with a pair of scissors on the perineum (the piece of flesh between the vagina and the anus) either at an angle or else down the midline. It is still very common practice for the majority of mothers, especially with their first birth, to be given episiotomies routinely. In some hospitals all mothers have them. Statistics in Great Britain range between 30 and 90 per cent.

The cut is usually made when the baby's head 'crowns' in the second stage of labour. The flesh around the mother's perineum is injected with a local anaesthetic to prevent her feeling any pain from the incision. After the birth the cut has to be stitched and this can take an hour or more. It is done with a curved needle and a local anaesthetic is again used.

In fact very few women actually need episiotomies (probably less than 4 per cent). It is the only surgical operation performed on a woman without her previous consent.

During pregnancy the soft tissues of the perineum 'ripen' so that they are capable of stretching open to allow the baby's head to pass through for birth. The reason usually given for routine episiotomy is that it prevents tearing, but in fact a natural tear heals much better. Many women don't tear at all, but if a tear does occur – and it is a natural hazard of birth – it is more superficial than an episiotomy which cuts through muscles, nerve tissue and skin.

For an episiotomy to be performed the mother has to lie down with her feet up, often in stirrups. This can completely ruin the final moments of the birth. If she is standing, squatting or kneeling her pelvis and perineum are open and relaxed and there is no need to intervene surgically in order to help her baby out. In its rightful place episiotomy should be used only as an emergency procedure when a baby is at risk and needs to be born quickly. Before booking to have her baby in hospital your partner could find out the policy on episiotomy. If she is free to refuse one and wishes to do so this should be recorded on her notes ahead of time.

Drugs used in childbirth

At one time it was thought that the placenta acted as a barrier, filtering out substances which could be harmful to the baby. Research has now established that in fact anything the mother consumes will pass through the placenta from her bloodstream into her baby's circulation. Therefore pain-relieving drugs commonly used in childbirth will pass through the placenta and affect the unborn baby in the womb.

When birth is active the need for painkillers is greatly reduced. However, these drugs are used so widely that it is important to have some knowledge of their advantages and disadvantages. Before choosing the place of birth your partner could find out which methods of pain relief are available even though, in all likelihood she won't even think of taking pain-relieving drugs.

It is important that the mother should *consent* to taking a drug in labour. You can help by knowing the subject and being available to help her if she ends up needing or wanting to choose some form of pain relief. The following are the most commonly used.

PETHEDINE

Pethedine is a narcotic used as an analgesic (painkiller). It is usually given as an intra-muscular injection and takes ten to twenty minutes to take effect. In some hospitals it is offered routinely to all women in labour. When Pethedine was first used it was given in a dose of 25 milligrams and this has increased over the years so that these days often a dose is between 100 and 150 milligrams. As one of the drug's side effects is nausea it is often mixed with an anti-emetic, which makes the mother very drowsy. In practice Pethedine is more effective as a muscle relaxant than as a painkiller and it can sometimes help to relax the cervix.

Some women feel very sleepy after taking Pethedine and find it difficult to cope with the contractions, particularly if it is given too late in the labour. If the mother is given Pethedine the drug will pass through to her baby in the same dosage. It is now well known that large quantities of Pethedine have a depressing effect on a baby's breathing response, so that at birth the child may need to be given oxygen and resuscitated. The baby may also then be given an anti-depressant as an antidote. Pethedine can also affect the baby's sucking reflex. This can last for some weeks after the birth and cause difficulties in establishing breastfeeding. The early contact between mother and baby is therefore disturbed. The side effects of Pethedine are so marked that many paediatricians today prefer it not to be used. Some women report that they found it helpful but usually they have taken a small dose of no more than 50 milligrams and this before 7 centimetres' dilation in the first stage.

The majority of women react to Pethedine by being less in control of the labour. With their perceptions dimmed they are less able to participate themselves. Their dependance on the attendants therefore increases as does the need for intervention.

GAS AND AIR (ENTONOX)

This is a mixture of 70 per cent nitrous oxygen and 30 per cent oxygen and is similar to the 'laughing gas' used by dentists. It comes in a tank which is kept beside the labour bed and the mother can use the mask to inhale the gas herself.

The advantage of Entonox is that one can inhale as much as necessary and then stop. Women who find it helpful often say that it has the effect of lifting one above what is happening. If used in large quantities or continuously through the first stage, the effects can be very unpleasant causing the mother to feel sleepy and out of control. It seems to be most effective when used at the end of the first stage to help the mother to cope with the most difficult contractions just before dilation is complete.

To use

The mother should place the mask over her nose just as she feels the contraction begin, then inhale and exhale deeply two or three times, putting the mask down before the peak of the contraction. This will give her mild pain relief within a few seconds which will last for about a minute. The effects are not cumulative. The gas will of course also reach the baby in the uterus, but it is cleared from his system when breathing is established after the birth.

TRILENE

This is similar to Entonox but it does have a cumulative effect on both mother and baby causing drowsiness and a drugged, nightmarish feeling if used in large quantities. The effects last for twenty minutes or so.

EPIDURALS

With this form of analgesia an anaesthetic fluid, similar to that used in dentistry, is injected into the epidural space surrounding the spinal cord. An epidural takes about half an hour to insert.

The mother is asked to curl up on her left side in a foetal position or to sit up and lean forward. A local anaesthetic is then injected into the skin around the lumbar area of her back to deaden sensation. The anaesthetic is then injected between two vertebrae into the epidural space. The needle is withdrawn and a thin plastic catheter left in, in case the anaesthetic needs to be topped up. This is taped in position on the mother's back and connected to a little cup attached to her shoulder where the top-up is given. This prevents the need for another injection.

When an epidural works, the mother will loose all sensation (pleasant as well as painful!) from the waist down and pain relief is total. A Caesarean section can be done using epidural anaesthesia and has the advantage of the mother being able to remain fully conscious (see page 145).

Once the mother has been given an epidural she is immobilized and will probably be attached to an electronic heart monitor. Sometimes epidurals don't work, giving only partial pain relief or anaesthesia down one side only.

An epidural reduces the muscular function of the uterus, causing weaker contractions so that there is a 20 per cent greater chance of the baby needing to be delivered with the help of forceps. The mother's bladder is affected too and needs to be emptied with a catheter during labour.

Epidurals lower the mother's blood pressure, which may be an advantage when blood pressure is unusually high, but normally a sudden drop may make the mother feel nauseous and faint. It will also affect the baby, reducing the supply of blood and oxygen reaching the uterus and placenta (see page 141). If the dura, the membrane surrounding the spinal cord, is accidentally scratched or punctured, the effect is complete spinal anaesthesia, which is heavier and can result in severe headaches which last several days after the birth.

Much research on the effects of an epidural on the baby still needs to be done. They reach the baby's system within minutes but do not affect the breathing or sucking reflex as does Pethedine. Doris Haire, a leading American expert on drugs, is convinced from her investigations and research that epidurals may well be the cause of the great increase in neurological disorders amongst children in the USA, as the anaesthetic enters the brain and nerve cells of the baby which are developing rapidly at the time of birth and for several months thereafter.*

Because of its attendant risks, the routine use of an epidural for normal births is not advisable. In circumstances where total pain relief or a Caesarean section is necessary, however, or if the first stage is over-prolonged and difficult, an epidural may be very helpful. It is important for the mother to be examined internally to check dilation before having an epidural. If given too late in labour she is unlikely to be able to push the baby out herself without help. If requested the anaesthetist can arrange to insert the epidural between 4–7 centimetres' dilation and to give as mild a dose as possible so that the mother can still feel the contractions a little and may be able to push effectively herself in the second stage.

GENERAL ANAESTHETIC

This is used for a Caesarean section. On the rare occasion that a baby becomes distressed in labour and needs to be born immediately a general anaesthetic is usually given. The mother is given an injection of Pentothol, which brings unconsciousness within seconds. She is then held under general anaesthesia with gas until the baby is delivered and will come round within half an hour or so of the birth.

* See Doris Haire, 'The Cultural Warping of Childbirth', in *Environmental Child Health*, Vol. 19, pp. 17–91, June 1973.

Birth at home

In many ways a home birth is the ideal setting for an active birth. From the mother's point of view, she is on her own ground and has complete freedom to move from room to room, change positions, relax in the shower or bath, listen to music or do whatever she wishes. She is the only person giving birth, as opposed to being one more patient in the labour ward, it is her day and those around her can give her all their time and attention. She is in control of her own labour and can have people of her own choosing around to help and encourage her. If she is hoping for a natural birth she may find it easier to avoid drugs and intervention in her weaker moments if she remains outside the hospital environment.

Sometimes your doctor may be the best person to advise you on this, depending on his or her general attitude to home birth. There is no reason why a healthy woman with a normal pregnancy should not have her baby at home, whether it is her first or her fifth. Being over thirty is not a reason for having a baby in hospital.

For many women having a baby is an intensely spiritual and sexual experience. In her own home, surrounded by familiar objects, she can abandon herself more easily to her deepest instincts, drop her inhibitions and surrender to the powerful forces and emotions which make this one of the richest and most momentous experiences of her life. I have noticed, when I have had the privilege to be present at a home birth, how creative women and their partners can be in their own setting. Many women discover a 'birth dance' (see page 85), or find a song or sound that helps them. They would find it difficult to do this surrounded by the sterile hospital ward and unfamiliar staff.

Many fathers too, feel far more comfortable and at ease at home and find it easier to tune in to their partner's needs. When birth is active the father can participate fully in the labour and birth more easily so that the couple is in fact giving birth together as a team. Some fathers actually want to 'catch' the baby as it is born and many enjoy cutting the umbilical cord themselves. At a home birth it is possible to bath the baby in warm water soon after the birth. Many couples view the birth of their child as part of their sexual love for each other, the fruit of the lovemaking that created their baby. They often enjoy a close and tender physical contact throughout the labour and need intimacy and freedom to express themselves without inhibition.

With a home birth it is much easier to have continuity of care and you will probably both have many opportunities to discuss important issues with your doctor or midwife before the birth. From their point of view they have time to get to know both father and mother as well as the rest of the family and will find it easier to help when the time comes.

When birth takes place at home it occurs as part of family life. This is particularly helpful when there is an older child or children. They can be present at the birth and will not have to experience a long separation from one or both parents at the same time.

The creation of a family or the birth of a new member of it is a time of emotional change and evolution which deeply affects everyone concerned. When birth takes place at home the sequence of events unfolds naturally and the normal continuity of life remains undisturbed, making it easier for all involved to accept and adjust to the new situation. A home birth is particularly rewarding in the hours and days after the birth. The couple or family and new baby can remain together, sleep together, bathe together and so on, as they please, getting to know each other in their own time. The mother, for her part, does not have to be isolated from her family at this very special time.

The birth of a baby generates a wonderful 'high energy' in a home. It is a time of celebration and often a euphoria and a blissful, rare feeling of peace descends on the household which lasts for a week or more after the birth. In hospital this feeling is often lost or obliterated by hospital routine and overcrowding. There are, then, many advantages to a home birth. It is, however, important to have good ante-natal care, to be well prepared and to be sure that this is the right choice for you both.

The safety issue

There is no possible way that birth can be without risk. Statistics and research show that home birth is as safe, if not safer, than hospital birth. Holland has the lowest perinatal mortality rate in Europe and yet the majority of women there give birth at home.

However, what is important is to assess whether your partner will be safer and better off in hospital or at home. The vast majority of babies are born safely. The mother's own feelings and instincts are the most important guide, however, and here are some good reasons for having a baby in hospital.

A previous complicated birth
If the reason for the previous complications are likely to effect this birth, for instance if the mother has a small pelvic capacity or has had a previous Caesarean section.

Placenta praevia
If the placenta is lying in the lower part of the uterus and covering the cervix. There is a danger that the placenta will separate before the baby is born, so usually a Caesarean section is needed.

Premature birth
If the baby is more than three weeks early it may be very small and need incubation and paediatric care.

Pre-eclampsia
This occurs in about 5 per cent of all women in late pregnancy. (The statistics are far lower if ante-natal preparation, diet and exercise are good.)

The early symptoms are a rise in blood pressure and fluid retention. If these symptoms occur together, the mother has mild pre-eclampsia. With treatment this condition can improve, but if it advances, another symptom – that of protein in the mother's urine – will probably develop. If all these symptoms are present together then the mother has pre-eclampsia. Even though she may still be feeling well, there is a danger that the placenta may fail to nourish the baby and premature birth is possible.

The general health of the mother
If the mother is very overweight or underweight, anaemic, in poor health, has diabetes or persistent high blood pressure. (A slight rise in blood pressure towards the end of pregnancy is perfectly normal and does not indicate the need for hospital birth but does call for careful observation in case it goes up.)

Haemorrhage
If there is a previous history of haemorrhage.

Rh negative blood
If a woman has Rh negative blood it is quite safe for her to have a home birth unless she has a positive antibody test.

Breech presentation/Twins

If the baby is in a breech position or if there are twins, then successful delivery depends on the skill and experience of the attendants.

Arranging a home birth can sometimes be problematic. If so, contact one of the groups listed on page 165 for help and advice.

Partners in hospital

These days it is generally accepted in hospital that either the father of the baby or one other partner will accompany a woman in labour. In some hospitals the mother is able to bring more than one person along, for example her husband and a friend, ante-natal teacher or other member of her family. Some hospitals are now experimenting with family birthing rooms where even other siblings could be present, but there are not many of these.

Find out beforehand what the hospital policy is on this matter and if possible have written confirmation that you intend to be there attached to the mother's notes to avoid disappointment at the last minute.

In a busy labour ward the staff generally don't have much time to look after partners and you are unlikely to be offered a meal, even though you may be there for many hours. Go well prepared with food and anything you might need as you may not want to leave your partner alone for very long. There is usually a 'fathers' room' with comfortable chairs or a couch, a tea and coffee machine and pay phone for your use.

Depending on what is provided by the hospital, there are a few things you can take with you which will be helpful in labour.

* A large, clean floor cushion or beanbag is indispensable in the conventional labour room as it provides the mother with the extra support she needs for kneeling and can help you too. With the aid of a large cushion and four or five pillows you can adapt a delivery bed to a much more useful piece of furniture.
* A natural sponge and two towelling face cloths are very useful for refreshing the mother between contractions.
* A picnic for yourself which includes some honey, red grape juice or apple juice for your partner (see page 81).
* Cash for the pay phone and coffee machine.

Active birthing rooms

Many hospitals throughout the UK are trying to accommodate couples who want to have an active birth by creating a birthing room. This differs from the conventional hospital room in that it is more like home, with a low platform or bed and is furnished like an ordinary bedroom. In some hospitals there is a wooden birthing stool or perhaps a mattress on the floor.

Michel Odent, in his hospital in Pithiviers in France, has created the ideal birthing room of this sort. He emphasizes the need for an atmosphere in which both the mother and her partner can feel completely at ease. He recommends the use of semi-darkness to help the mother to be more instinctive and to release any inhibitions. Adjoining the birthing room there is a bathroom with a round pool of water, rather like a large children's paddling pool, in which the mother and sometimes her partner too, can remain for several hours. Often when the labour is long, painful or difficult, relaxing in warm water can make all the difference to the woman giving birth. Sometimes the labour progresses so well that the baby is born in the pool.

7 The unexpected

Well over 90 per cent of all active births are likely to be uncomplicated and straightforward. However, every pregnancy and labour is an unknown adventure and anyone may experience unexpected problems or need obstetric intervention. Ultimately the most important thing is to have a healthy mother and baby.

It is wise, when preparing yourselves for an active birth, to spend some time considering the possibility of an unexpected complication arising, either in late pregnancy or during the labour itself. In this chapter most of the problems which could occur are listed together, which may prove to be frightening to the reader. Do remember that only one or two of these, if any, are likely to happen to your partner and in the unlikely event that they do, it is to your advantage to approach the situation with some knowledge, and common understanding. Even the most difficult birth can turn out to be a rewarding and moving experience.

Complications in late pregnancy

BLEEDING

It is quite common for very slight bleeding, known as 'spotting', to occur and this is generally nothing to worry about, though it is important to inform your birth attendants.

Just before labour starts there is often a 'show' of blood, which is the discharge of the plug of mucus which sealed the cervix. This too is perfectly normal. Any bleeding which is more than spotting or a show could indicate a possible problem and should be reported immediately to your midwife, doctor or hospital. In the unlikely event of your partner experiencing acute, abnormal pain and/or a steady stream of period-like bleeding, she should be taken to hospital immediately. This happens very rarely and could be caused by premature separation of the placenta. In this case an emergency Caesarean may be necessary.

OEDEMA (swelling or fluid retention)

Many women, particularly in hot weather, experience fluid retention towards the end of pregnancy. It is especially noticeable in the face, hands, and feet, which appear slightly swollen and puffy. This is quite normal and will disappear after the birth. Homoeopathic treatment can be effective and it can also help to cut out salt from the diet and to rest a lot. If the swelling increases or happens suddenly it may be a sign of toxaemia (see below).

HIGH BLOOD PRESSURE (hypertension)

A rise in blood pressure towards the end of pregnancy is quite common. It can be a sign of pre-eclampsia (see below) when combined with other symptoms, but more often it is caused by excitement, fear or other emotional reasons as the day of birth approaches. A busy ante-natal clinic can often cause a mother's blood pressure to rise, particularly if she is stressed by waiting for a long time. Resting in bed can help to reduce blood pressure and homoeopathic treatment is often effective.

PRE-ECLAMPSIA (toxaemia)

When a woman in late pregnancy has high blood pressure combined with fluid retention and protein in her urine she has a condition known as pre-eclampsia. This affects only a small percentage of women and in its mild form can be reduced or removed by bed rest. Sometimes sedatives are suggested and homoeopathic treatment can be effective.

It is often very difficult for a woman with mild pre-eclampsia to accept the fact that she needs some form of treatment as she may be feeling and looking very well. This condition does, however, need careful attention. If it worsens, it may mean that the placenta is not functioning as well as normal and the baby could be endangered in which case it might be safer outside the womb. Obstetric intervention is often advisable here.

It is possible to test the efficiency of the placenta by measuring the amount of oestrogen in the mother's blood and or urine (oestriol test). The best way to help your partner is to try to allow her complete rest and peace of mind and to free her from any household responsibilities while offering her your encouragement and support.

LOW-LYING PLACENTA OR PLACENTA PRAEVIA

Here the placenta is set low in the uterus rather than up at the top. It occurs in approximately one out of two hundred pregnancies and can be seen on an ultrasound scan. Often this presents no problem as the placenta rises up in the last weeks of pregnancy as the uterus grows and a normal birth is possible. Sometimes, however, the placenta may partially or completely cover the cervix. In this case there is a danger that it may separate from the wall of the uterus before the baby is born. This would mean that the baby would lose its life-line for food and oxygen and be in danger of death from asphyxia and it has to be delivered by Caesarean section.

ABRUPTIO PLACENTA

This occurs very rarely and means that the placenta completely separates from the wall of the uterus before the baby is born. The cause is often unknown and the symptoms are bleeding or severe pain and hardness in the abdomen. Immediate medical attention in hospital is necessary.

THE POSITION OF THE BABY

As the time of labour approaches, the position in which the baby presents itself for birth becomes important. Most babies present head down and feet up with the head 'engaged' in the pelvic brim some weeks before the birth (anterior position). If the baby's head does not engage during labour, then a problem of pelvic disproportion or position is a possibility.

If the baby is in an unusual position the mother's instinctive knowledge of how best to position herself to help her baby out, often has amazing results. When the baby is lying in a posterior position, the kneeling positions combined with squatting are helpful. Often, if the mother rotates her hips it will help the baby to rotate through the birth canal. If the baby is lying breech (see page 33) the supported standing squat is recommended.

If the mother does not succeed to find a way to deliver her baby, then the help of forceps or a Caesarean section may be necessary.

LATE FOR DATES

Very often a normal pregnancy lasts longer than the average estimated due date. Two or even three weeks overdue is not uncommon, particularly in women who have long menstrual cycles. Many birth attendants are not concerned if your partner should go over her due date. However in some hospitals the policy is to wait seven to fourteen days or less and then to induce the birth.

If your partner is being pressurized to have the birth induced this can cause considerable stress. It may help to find out whether this is the general policy of the doctor or hospital concerned and to ask detailed questions as to why induction is recommended. She could also ask for an ultrasound scan and an oestriol test to assess the size and position of the baby and the placental function. Generally, if these present no problems and there are no other medical indications, she is quite safe to wait for nature to take its course.

If induction is recommended your partner will need to weigh up the risks involved in inducing the birth and compare these with the risks of waiting. You can be supportive by accompanying her on her visits to the doctor or to hospital and by encouraging her to ask questions and request adequate tests. You can also help her to relax and forget about it by taking her out and perhaps enjoying some good wine together. If labour is imminent, making love can be one of the best ways to get it started.

WATERS BREAKING EARLY

Sometimes the membranes can rupture before labour starts. This can happen hours or even days before there are any contractions. Though this is quite normal and is not a sign of anything going wrong, the waters do provide a barrier to any bacteria that may enter the uterus and cause an infection. Once the sac is broken there is a slightly increased risk of infection to mother and baby. Occasionally the waters break a few weeks before the due date and in this case the prematurity of the baby may be another risk. Sometimes the sac of membranes can break or leak and then reseal and stay resealed for weeks. However, if the birth is imminent and the baby's head has already engaged, there is generally no harm in waiting twelve to twenty-four hours for nature to take its course. Your partner will be less exposed to infection in her own home where she is used to the bacteria than in a hospital ward. Your doctor may suggest antibiotic cover or alternatively if she prefers to avoid antibiotics your partner could take garlic capsules and Vitamin C to prevent infection. This will have a natural antibiotic effect without harming mother or baby. She should take seven to eight garlic capsules and 1 gram of Vitamin C every two or three hours until labour starts.

If the baby's head has not engaged, there is some danger of the cord prolapsing (see page 144) and in this case it is best for the mother to be in hospital as a precaution.

In some hospitals induction is suggested after six hours if the contractions have not started and this can present you and your partner with a difficult dilemma if she is hoping to avoid an induced birth. It will then be necessary to consider all the risks involved (see page 120) and to weigh these up against the advice of your attendants which may conflict with your partner's wishes. A failed induction can result in an unnecessary Caesarean section.

Many women, therefore, prefer to wait, to take measures to prevent infection and to keep a careful check on the baby's heartbeat and their own temperature. If these are monitored every few hours and are normal then there is no infection present and it is usually quite all right for her to wait to go into labour. In this situation it can make all the difference if you know how to check the baby's heartbeat yourselves every few hours (see page 116) because your partner can then stay at home until labour starts and avoid any pressure from others to induce.

PREMATURE LABOUR

It is perfectly normal for some women to start labour two or three weeks before their expected due date. Labour is considered to be premature, however, when it occurs more than three weeks early. If your partner should experience strong contractions, with or without bleeding, she may have begun labour prematurely. It is easy none the less to confuse real labour with practice contractions that occur a few weeks before birth or when the baby's head engages in the pelvis.

If you think that your partner is in premature labour, give her a strong alcoholic drink such as whisky or brandy. This will suppress the contractions. Get her to lie down immediately and relax and send for your doctor. Often a few days in bed will prevent an early labour.

If premature labour is confirmed the baby may not yet be fully mature and may be small and vulnerable to complications, possibly needing special care in hospital. Not quite yet ready for the outside world the baby may need help to keep warm and to breathe and it may be jaundiced and more susceptible to infections.

It can be quite distressing for you and your partner to see your baby in an intensive care unit, attached to tubes and wires and isolated in an incubator. It is, however, reassuring to know that these days most premature babies grow up none the worse for wear! Such a birth can come as quite a shock and the first days and weeks can be quite a stressful time for both parents.

In some enlightened hospitals premature babies are kept in an incubator which is placed beside the mother's bed. More usually the baby will be in a special intensive care ward while the mother is in a different post-natal ward. Both mothers and fathers are encouraged, in some hospitals, to handle and care for their babies as soon as possible. Partners can play an important role in this situation, helping to keep open a line of communication between mother and baby. Even though a baby is in an incubator, your presence and that of the mother is even more important. Encouraging and helping your partner to breastfeed her baby will help them both. A premature baby needs the best possible nutrition and protection from infection which is ideally provided by breastmilk.

When a birth is premature it is more difficult to begin breastfeeding. It may take a few days before the milk supply comes in and your partner will need extra encouragement to persevere through early difficulties. As soon as it is possible your baby will benefit from as much holding and body contact as you can manage between you.

Surprise birth

If your partner should go into labour unexpectedly and you find yourself alone with no time to get help the following suggestions may be useful.

1   First of all relax if you can. When birth is so rapid, nature is

usually at its most efficient and by simply allowing things to evolve, problems are very unlikely.

2   Wash your hands thoroughly if there is time.

3   Attend to your partner, making her comfortable and helping her to relax. If her contractions are very strong and rapid suggest that she use the all-fours position as this will help her to feel in control and slow down the contractions a little. Give her a cushion or beanbag to kneel against if possible. Spend a few minutes relaxing and breathing together.

4   Once your partner is relaxed, try to warm the room as the baby is used to body temperature and can chill easily.

5   Find a few clean towels, sheets or newspaper – whatever you have at hand – to keep the baby and mother warm. Place a clean towel on the floor between the mother's legs.

6   Get a bowl of warm water, a toilet roll and a bowl for the placenta.

7   Now get back to your partner and help her to concentrate on her breathing and the contractions, using massage and lots of encouragement if she needs it.

8   As the baby's head descends through the birth canal you will see first a round shape bulging around the vagina and then the head will appear through the opening. There is nothing for you to do apart from waiting for the uterus to do its work and keeping your hands nearby, ready to catch the baby who may come out very rapidly or else slowly over several contractions.

   Allow the baby's head to hang down naturally as it emerges and gravity will help to ensure perfect rotation. Once the head is out, first one shoulder, then the other and finally the whole body will slither out.

9   Hold the baby with your hand palm up under its chest with the face downwards to allow the fluids to drain.

10   Place the baby, again face downwards, on a clean sheet or towel on the floor for a few moments and then help your partner to sit down and pick up her baby. Do not cut the cord.

11   Both of you can now relax and enjoy the baby! Make sure that the mother is sitting really upright to facilitate perfect contact between her and the baby and that they are both warm.

   Encourage your partner to start breastfeeding as the suckling of the baby will stimulate the uterus to contract and expel the placenta.

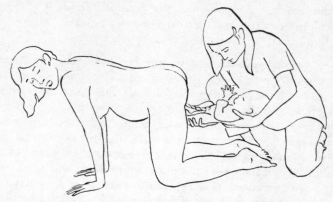

12　If the placenta is coming out ask your partner to squat over a bowl and keep the placenta beside her without cutting the cord.

13　Give her a drink of warm milk and honey, or tea as she will probably be a little shocked if the birth was very rapid.

14　After a while the mother could squat over a bowel of warm water to wash her genital area to prevent infection. Place a clean towel or sanitary pad between her legs.

15　Contact your doctor or midwife.

Complications in labour

FOETAL DISTRESS

The baby in the womb becomes distressed when he is not getting enough oxygen. This can be caused by a very long labour, problems with the functioning of the cord or placenta, or else from conditions in the mother such as pre-eclampsia. Perhaps the most common cause of foetal distress in labour is the use of the recumbent position, as this impedes the mother's circulation and therefore the flow of blood to and from the placenta.

Signs of foetal distress

★　Prolonged irregularity of the baby's heartbeat which could be slower or faster than it should be.

★　Meconium staining of the amniotic fluid. If the baby lacks oxygen in labour, the anal sphincter tends to relax and meconium (a dark green, sticky fluid which is the baby's first bowel

movement) is passed into the amniotic fluid. The normally colourless water will then turn brown or green.
★   Abnormally vigorous movements of the baby.

When two such indications of distress come together, the chances are that the baby is in trouble but it is not uncommon for one sign to occur and for the baby to be perfectly all right. A change of position will often help the heartbeat to return to normal. If, however, it drops below 100 beats per minute then the baby needs to be born as soon as possible. If the mother is still in the first stage of labour this will mean an emergency Caesarean is necessary (see page 144). If she is in the second stage the standing squat position will help to get the baby born quickly or else an episiotomy (see page 124) may need to be done to get the baby out as fast as possible. Your partner may be given oxygen to inhale to help the baby.

Either during the birth or when it is in the womb the baby may inhale some of the amniotic fluid containing meconium into its lungs. This could cause irritation or difficulty in breathing. For this reason immediately after the birth the midwife will probably clean the baby's nose and mouth by suction before he starts to breathe.

When a baby becomes distressed in labour, it is of course an unexpected shock to all concerned and things seem to move incredibly quickly as measures are taken to help the baby. You may find yourself feeling both worried and helpless as the midwife or hospital staff swing into action with no time to explain anything. The best thing you can do is to trust in their skills and efficiency and help to support your partner through these tense and trying moments.

PROLONGED FIRST STAGE

Labour can sometimes be very slow, progressing hardly at all over several hours even though your partner may be experiencing strong and frequent contractions. In some cases the contractions can cease completely or slow down for a while. There can be many causes for this. Often these are emotional and the woman needs to find her way of surrendering to what is happening in her body. It can be very disappointing to have prepared for months for an active birth, to be fitter and in better health than ever and then to find that the labour does not progress as fast or easily as expected. The reasons could vary from a very deep-seated psychological block, a previous trauma or negative experience to a straightforward physiological problem, such as the position of the baby or the size of the mother's pelvis.

You can help to avoid an unexpected emotional problem by making the most of the months of pregnancy to clear the air, talking with your partner and seeking professional help if necessary. Sometimes the mother needs to express deep feelings which she has been unable to release before she can let go, trust herself and those around her and give birth.

In this situation, as her partner you need to be creative to find a way to get things going. If the midwife does not suspect that there is a physiological cause one of the following suggestions may help.

* A warm bath or shower.
* A change of environment, perhaps a walk outside or into another room.
* A change of position.
* Something light to eat.
* A rest or sleep where you are left alone together to relax and forget about it.

FORCEPS OR VENTOUSE DELIVERY

When upright and squatting positions are used in labour and birth the number of births in which help is needed to get the baby out is drastically reduced by the help of gravity and an increased pelvic capacity. However, on rare occasions, help is needed.

Forceps
These look rather like curved metal salad spoons with a hole in the middle. If forceps are to be used the mother is either given an epidural or a local anaesthetic injection to numb the birth outlet.

An episiotomy is done to enlarge the opening and the forceps are inserted, one on either side of the baby's head and fastened together so that they cradle it firmly. The physician can then use the forceps to turn or lift the baby's head down the birth canal in harmony with the contractions from the uterus. The baby may have marks or bruises from the forceps but these disappear soon after the birth. Homoeopathic remedies such as Arnica will help the mother and baby to recover from any bruising or shock.

Ventouse or vacuum extraction
This works like a miniature vacuum cleaner which is attached to the

baby's head to help him out. There may be a swelling on his head for a day or two afterwards! Unless the baby is distressed and needs to be born immediately, it is well worth while trying to avoid the use of intervention by a change of position, immersion in water, or by relaxing and waiting for a really strong urge to get the baby born.

CAESAREAN BIRTH

A Caesarean birth is when the baby is delivered through a surgical incision in the mother's abdomen and uterus and circumstances occasionally arise in which it is the best course of action for the mother and/or the baby.

If you have been expecting a trouble-free natural birth the news that a Caesarean is necessary can come as a considerable shock. Sometimes you may have days or weeks of warning, giving you and your partner time to accept the situation and choose the attendants and type of anaesthesia to be used. On the other hand it may become apparent during labour that things are not progressing as they should and the decision to do a Caesarean might be made very quickly if the baby becomes distressed in the womb. In this case, you will have to adjust rapidly to the new situation.

Foetal distress (see page 141) is the commonest reason for a Caesarean section. This severe lack of oxygen to the baby can be caused by several things.

Compression of the umbilical cord

This occurs extremely rarely and means that the flow of blood to the baby, and therefore his supply of oxygen, is restricted or blocked. The reason for this could be that the cord has descended into the vagina ahead of the baby (prolapse of the cord). In this case, which occurs only in approximately one out of a thousand births, the baby's head may put pressure on the cord or it may go into spasm in the vagina. If so, the baby needs to be born immediately as its lifeline is physically blocked. The cord sometimes becomes blocked if it is wound too tightly around the baby's neck, although usually if this happens it is not compressed and the baby is quite all right.

Failure of the placenta to function in labour

This is evident when the baby's heartbeat develops an abnormal pattern due to the shortage of oxygen. In its most severe form the placenta could separate from the uterus partially or completely (see page 136).

Failure to progress in labour
There could be many reasons for this (see page 142).

Abnormal presentation of the baby
Occasionally a baby can be lying crosswise in the uterus and cannot be turned. Sometimes a difficult posterior or breech presentation may require a Caesarean.

The shape of the pelvis
Most babies are made to measure to their mother's pelvic capacity. Occasionally, however, a baby is too big to fit through or the mother's pelvis is unusually small or irregular in shape.

These are some of the main causes for a Caesarean. Every situation is unique though and it is important for you and your partner to have a detailed explanation from the obstetrician, if possible before, but certainly after the operation. In particular you should ask whether these reasons will affect your partner if she has another baby.

Elective Caesarean
If you know in advance that your partner is to have a Caesarean, then she has the advantage of choosing which sort of anaesthetic she would prefer. She could have a general anaesthetic, in which case she will be unconscious whilst the operation is done and for a while afterwards. Alternatively, many hospitals now do Caesareans under epidural anaesthesia (see page 127). This has the advantage of the mother being able to remain fully conscious and so having immediate contact with her baby. This method is becoming increasingly popular and for many couples it provides a very satisfactory solution. Fathers are often invited to attend and if you should wish to do so, do discuss the procedure with the obstetrician in detail beforehand.

Some women, who know that for various reasons their baby will be born by Caesarean, still choose to wait to go into spontaneous labour and experience the first stage partially or completely before the operation. This has the advantage of ensuring the exact maturity of the baby. Also many experts feel that the massage of the contracting uterus is important for the baby and that the experience of labour, even if briefer than normal, is still significant to the mother in terms of her relationship with the child. If the need for a Caesarean arises as an emergency then there is no time to insert an epidural and a general anaesthetic is used.

How you can help

Either during the birth itself or in the hours afterwards your partner will find deep breathing a helpful way to relax and focus her mind. Before, during or after the operation you can support her by concentrating your attention on her, encouraging her and helping her to stay calm and centred. It can make all the difference to her if she is able to share her emotions and can feel you are working as a team.

You can also help the baby by standing in for your partner until she is able to take care of him or her. The attendants can pass the baby to you as soon as he is born. You can hold the baby and welcome him, shielding his eyes from harsh light and standing nearby when he is examined. If your partner is conscious you can ensure that she sees and holds her baby immediately after birth.

Women who have prepared for an active birth by stretching usually recover from a Caesarean very quickly. The operation is a major one, however, and in the days immediately after the birth, your partner will take time to recover from the effects of the anaesthetic and will be in considerable discomfort from the wound. She will need extra help to lift, care for and feed her baby. Seven to ten days after the birth she will be able to return home but will need help with domestic chores and caring for the rest of the family, as her strength will be limited and she will require plenty of rest to recuperate. It will take her perhaps several months to feel strong and energetic again. By planning and preparing for these days ahead of time you can help her to have a relaxed recovery and a successful start to breastfeeding her baby.

Problems of the third stage of labour

RETAINED PLACENTA

The placenta is usually expelled from the uterus within an hour of the birth. Very occasionally it fails to separate and may need to be removed manually. In this case the mother can be given anaesthesia or an epidural. Homoeopathic remedies are sometimes helpful. The use of upright postures in labour and birth is the best way to avoid this sort of problem.

HAEMORRHAGE

This is excessive bleeding from the uterus after the birth. It usually occurs because the muscles of the uterus lose their tension and cannot contract sufficiently to stop the bleeding at the spot where the placenta has separated from the uterus wall. When birth is active and medication is not used unnecessarily, this is very unlikely.

A woman can haemorrhage after the birth or any time during the first day. Bleeding after the birth is quite normal as the uterus sheds its blood-rich lining but a haemorrhage entails the loss of at least 500 millilitres (2 cups) of blood.

To treat a haemorrhage the mother is usually placed flat on her back with her feet up. Her uterus is firmly massaged to stimulate the contractions and she is given an injection of syntocinon to make the uterus contract. She is also usually given a blood transfusion to help make up for the loss of blood. If she has lost a lot of blood she will probably be very pale and weak until her fluid balance is restored.

Abnormality

Every parent-to-be will probably consider at some time the possibility of their baby being born with some defect, handicap or abnormality. Some people experience much anxiety about this and in the vast majority of cases their fears turn out to be unfounded. Abnormalities are very rare, but they do occur and it is realistic to approach parenthood having thought of how one might cope with such a situation, unlikely though it is.

Abnormalities can occur in the formation of part of the baby's body, such as the spine, as with spina-bifida, or in the digestive or circulatory systems.

Today, in our modern hospitals, help is readily available and physiological problems can often be improved or cured surgically or with some other form of treatment. Most abnormalities are treatable and there are also usually helpful support organizations.

Very rarely a baby may have Down's Syndrome or be mentally retarded or have some defect of sight or hearing. Whatever the problem is, you are both bound to undergo a range of intense reactions and feelings as you adjust your expectations to the reality and problems of the moment.

Stillbirth

Although stillbirth is rare, it does nevertheless occur and it is certainly worth giving some thought to how you both might cope with such a situation. Sometimes the causes of death are known but not always. In either case death always comes as a shock and is a painful experience to integrate into everyday life.

If the baby dies some days or weeks before labour starts your partner may have to await the labour knowing that she will give birth to a dead baby. This is inevitably a very difficult experience but even in this situation it may still be worthwhile for her to have a spontaneous, active birth. One mother I know who did so told me later that this was the most positive part of the experience. She felt that she had learned how to give birth and indeed this knowledge came in very handy with her two subsequent pregnancies. Her partner, who accompanied her on all three occasions, tells me how it helped them both to go through the first birth together, bringing them into closer and deeper communication. He feels that this created a stronger foundation for the two healthy babies they now have.

Sometimes a baby may die during the labour or shortly afterwards. In this case it is best if your attendants tell you both the truth as it happens. Your partner will cope better with the reality, however painful, than with confusion and deceit.

Many professionals feel that it is a good idea for the parents of a stillborn baby to see and hold their baby after the birth. (Modern astrologers consider the period of life in the womb until gestation to be one third of the lifetime of a human being.) Even if a baby dies at birth both parents, and the mother in particular, have a profound relationship with their child and the experience of loss will be deep and take time to accept. You are bound to experience feelings of shock, anger and guilt and to go through a period of grief and mourning. This can last for several months to a year or more and can affect one's relationships both with friends and each other for some time.

As partner to a woman who has lost a baby, perhaps the best way you can help her is simply to be there to share her feelings and to listen to her as she makes the emotional adjustment. It can only help her to feel less alone and isolated if you express your own emotions to her. If you try to be too matter of fact she will probably think that you don't understand. It is not easy to find oneself with empty arms after months of preparing for a new baby and possibly after hours of labour. You are both bound to feel isolated and a victim of circumstance at first, but given time and freedom to express your feelings you will recover from and accept the loss.

It can be helpful to contact an organization such as the Stillbirth Association where you will have the opportunity to meet other people who have had similar experiences and you can obtain help and advice. Your doctor should have the address of the branch nearest to you.

8 After the birth

THE NEWBORN BABY

Immediately after birth a newborn baby probably does not resemble the ideal you have been imagining. His body will be quite wet, possibly covered in some blood from the rich lining of the uterus. The colour of the baby the moment after he is born can be slightly grey or blue. As soon as he begins to breathe a few seconds later, his body will become pink. The skin of the baby may be quite wrinkled and could be covered with a layer of a white, creamy substance called vernix. This protects the baby against the change in temperature and is also full of nutritious substances which the baby absorbs into its body. The vernix will have been absorbed into the baby's skin a few hours after birth. The head may be slightly pointed in shape. This is caused by the overlapping or moulding of the bones of the skull as the baby passes through the pelvic canal. Within a few hours the shape will become round again.

The baby will open his eyes and will be able to see everything around him. His length of focus at this stage is approximately that of the distance from his mother's face when held in her arms. The cooler air on his skin will stimulate the breathing reflex as he starts to inhale air for the first time. He will be able to smell and taste and will have a sucking reflex so that he is soon ready to find and make contact with his mother's breast. He is an exquisitely sensitive creature and at the same time quite strong and sturdy.

THE FIRST HOUR

If your partner has given birth actively without medication the baby will be extremely alert and sensitive to everything that is happening in the first hour or so after the birth. This hour is a very special time when the baby adjusts to the change from the dark, watery and confined space in the womb to new sights, sounds, smells, and sensations. Many of his vital functions start now, when no longer nourished by the placenta, he learns to breathe, digest and excrete independently.

In the hours and days that follow the baby will spend most of the time sleeping deeply or feeding. The way we welcome our newborn and the quality of our first contact, either between mother and baby or mother, father, and baby can significantly affect all of us in the years to come. A baby born naturally and welcomed lovingly into the world has the best possible start in life. Researchers have emphasized the importance of this first hour after birth and show how a good 'bonding' at this time between mother, baby and father can help relationships in the growing family. A mother who enjoys an undisturbed first contact with her baby has a good start in the ease with which she can communicate with her child. During this time it is helpful if the birth attendants withdraw and leave you all alone together for at least half an hour to give you a chance to welcome the baby.

In some situations it is impossible for mother and baby to enjoy this early contact in the ideal way (for instance, if the mother has a general anaesthetic or the baby needs to be resuscitated). What is most important is that the mother really loves her baby and she can always find ways to make up for the contact missed immediately after birth.

A good 'bonding' is facilitated if the mother sits completely upright while holding her baby. In this way the eye to eye, skin to skin, and mouth to nipple contact between them is perfect. If she needs support, try standing or sitting behind her. The baby will have a powerful instinct to find the nipple, known as a 'rooting reflex', and will probably want to start suckling at the breast within the first hour. This first sucking helps to facilitate successful breastfeeding and it also stimulates the mother's body to release the hormones which contract the uterus and expel the placenta. Early contact with the breast produces an intensification in the mother's feelings of pleasure in caring for her baby which consolidates the bond between them and reassures and comforts the baby. The warmth of the mother's breasts and body improves and stimulates the baby's breathing and thus helps to oxygenate the blood, ensuring the baby's physical wellbeing.

THE FIRST FEW DAYS

In the days which follow your partner will be intensely involved in getting to know her baby, learning to take care of him and understand his needs and signals. At the same time she will go through many physiological changes as she recovers from the birth, her body slowly returns to a non-pregnant state and breastfeeding is established. Emotionally she must adjust to the reality of being a mother and learn to include the new demands of motherhood in her daily life.

In these early days her energy is likely to be almost totally absorbed in learning to adapt to her baby's needs. The symbiotic relationship between them, which was present during pregnancy and birth, continues once the baby is born. Gradually a harmonious rhythm between mother and baby evolves which will become a normal part of family life. To start with, though, coping with all the many changes means that it is likely to be a very unsettled and emotional time.

For the father this period is equally demanding. You too will need to adjust to the reality of being a parent and to the inclusion of a new person into your family life and your relationship with your partner. She is likely to need your support, encouragement and love more than ever at this time and you may find yourself needing to spread your energy between being with her and the baby and being at work. If you are already a father you will probably have the important task of taking care of your other children and helping them to get to know and accept the new member of the family.

The easiest way to integrate all these changes into your life is to take the line of least resistance. Make the new baby the first priority and try to allow your partner to have the freedom to discover a natural rhythm between her needs and those of her baby. She will need to eat well and to get plenty of rest, sleeping when the baby sleeps and generally 'playing it by ear', allowing the baby to be her guide. You will find it easier to help her if you understand the changes she is going through.

PHYSIOLOGICAL CHANGES IN THE MOTHER

After the birth the mother's uterus will continue to contract each time the baby suckles and will gradually return to its pre-pregnant size and shape. This takes between four to six weeks. At first these contractions can be uncomfortable but after a few weeks they become pleasurable or unnoticable. Bleeding will continue for a few weeks after the birth like a long period, but will gradually lessen and then cease altogether. If your partner had a perineal tear or episiotomy and has had stitches, the wound will generally heal quite rapidly within the first fortnight.

BREASTFEEDING

In the first few days after the birth your partner's breasts will produce a syrupy yellow fluid known as 'colostrum' which is the first milk made by the breasts. It is richer than mature breast milk in that it contains more protein and has antibodies which protect the baby from infection. It is the ideal food for the first two days after birth and does not need to be supplemented with anything else. It also acts as a laxative, clearing and preparing the baby's digestive system.

On the third day after birth the mother's breasts will begin to produce the mature milk which is white, thinner and more watery than colostrum. This is usually a very intense experience and you can expect her to be extremely emotional and probably weepy on the day that the milk 'comes in'. Her breasts may become very hard and full and much larger in size. This is known as 'engorgement' and can be very uncomfortable. After a few days the supply of milk will adjust to the baby's appetite and the discomfort will pass. It can help to stand under a warm shower before your partner feeds the baby and to massage her breasts from under her arms towards the nipple or else for her to lie on her belly in a bath of warm water.

Breast milk is the ideal food for the baby, and so it is well worth while helping and encouraging your partner to persevere through any early difficulties. Many of these can be avoided by if she allows the baby to feed whenever he wants to for as long as the baby requires. Encourage your partner to feed the baby like a gypsy rather than by the clock, perhaps allowing him to fall asleep at the breast. This provides him with warmth and contact as well as food. Babies differ in their ways of feeding – some suck for five or ten minutes and are satisfied while others need to suck for hours.

Breastfeeding is a fundamental requirement for a child. A baby can survive and thrive without it but will have a better start in life if breastfed. Indeed, research has shown that breastfed babies walk, talk and develop quicker than those which have been bottlefed.

From conception onwards mother and baby form a biological unit. This continues after the birth. The intimacy that results from breastfeeding has reciprocal psycho–physiological benefits for both mother and child which are vitally important to their future relationship. This is the baby's first socializing experience and it forms a foundation for the future. As Ashley Montague describes in his book *Touching*, in the hours spent at the breast in his mother's arms the baby: 'touches with its hands, presses with its lips, looks at her for hours, gets pleasure, security, and fulfilment which forms the basis of the gentle satisfaction and pleasures we have throughout life.'

ACTIVE FATHERING

Many fathers, who share and actively help their partners during pregnancy and birth, enjoy a continuous involvement in the care and nurturing of their babies. Today we are no longer as deeply bound by sexual stereotypes in our definitions of parenthood and many couples choose to share the joys and responsibilities of parenting according to their talents and inclinations.

In supporting your partner through pregnancy and childbirth you will have begun a deep involvement, a partnership in parenthood, which can continue in the months and years that follow. Your enthusiasm can be a major factor in successful breastfeeding and you can help your partner immensely to enjoy her new role as a mother without feeling isolated. The period of infancy and the first years is a very special time in a child's life and indeed it passes very quickly. Your child will have the benefit of having two parents who are central to his or her development. You yourself have a wonderful opportunity to learn more about yourself in the hours spent caring for your baby. A young baby needs a lot of time and attention but the compensations are many and the child's marvellous innocence can help us discover new ways of viewing both ourselves and the world around us.

AFTER BIRTH BLUES

After the tremendous physical and emotional experience of the birth don't be surprised if you or your partner find yourselves feeling, at times, empty, depressed or exhausted. Many couples after an active birth also experience the opposite side of the coin – a kind of 'post-natal euphoria', a time of great happiness and joy which can last for several weeks. When birth is active and mother and baby do not suffer the effects of medication or disturbance of the natural processes, serious post-natal depression is rarely a problem. However, it is quite normal and understandable to go through a 'down' after the intensity and high energy of the birth.

During pregnancy your partner's body was flooded continuously with female hormones from the placenta. Once the birth is over and the placenta has been discarded she has to adjust to a complete hormonal change which will certainly affect her emotionally. It is very common for women to feel depressed or weepy, usually between the third and sixth day after the birth. You too are likely to feel exhausted or low at times, particularly if your partner and the baby are in hospital and you have to return home alone.

The best way to avoid these blues is to make sure you all have enough sleep and rest and to try, as far as is possible, not to disturb the natural continuity between mother and baby. Allow the baby's needs to take precedence at first. Try to spend plenty of time relaxing together and enjoying the new baby and let practicalities and housework take second place for a while.

THE BABY'S CORD

After the cord stops pulsating it is usually clamped or tied and cut about an inch away from the baby's navel. It will gradually dry up and fall off within the first week or so. Keep it dry and clean and try to prevent the baby's nappy from rubbing against it.

JAUNDICE

It is common for a baby to look slightly yellow, rather as if it has a suntan, for two or three days after the birth. When birth is unmedicated this is less likely to happen. Though this is called post-natal jaundice it bears no relation to the disease and is simply caused by a temporary excess of red blood cells in the baby's system. In the womb the baby needed these to handle its need for oxygen but after the birth they are not required and are broken down by the baby's body. A by-product of this breakdown is an excess of bilirubin which is deposited in the skin and causes the yellowish coloration.

The colostrum and first milk help to clear the system. Sunshine helps too so it is a good idea to place the baby naked in a warm spot in the sunlight for half-hour intervals, making sure his or her eyes are shaded. If the jaundice is more severe then the hospital or attendants may suggest that the baby needs to be treated under an ultra-violet lamp. This is, however, rarely necessary.

SLEEP

In the first few days after the birth the baby is alert and wide awake. After this he will sleep for long periods, waking up mainly to feed. The baby will have his own biorhythms which are likely to vary in the beginning until they settle into a more stable pattern. These differ from child to child. The baby may have a period of wakefulness at the same time every day, may need feeding every two or three hours throughout the twenty-four, or may have long sleep periods.

The parents of a newborn baby can find the change and disruption of their sleeping habits difficult to adapt to. It is a good idea for the mother to try to sleep whenever her baby does. If you need to go to work then it may help to have an extra bed in another room to avoid being disturbed if you are tired.

It is certainly less exhausting for all concerned if the baby sleeps right next to the mother, either in the same bed or in a basket or crib beside it. Many couples enjoy sleeping together in bed with their baby and this can help your partner to feed the baby at night without really having to wake up and get out of bed.

Always remember to place a newborn baby on his stomach to sleep so that any milk coming up will not choke him.

WHAT TO DO WHEN YOUR BABY CRIES

Usually a baby who cries is hungry. The baby may, however, want to be held, comforted, changed or simply need to express his feelings. Most babies have a fretful time of day. You and your partner will learn through trial and error how to understand your baby's signal.

A baby is also very much affected by the moods and emotions of others around him, particularly the mother. If she is tired, anxious, stressed or irritable the baby is likely to be restless too. At times like these you can help enormously by taking the baby away from the mother and giving them both a bit of space to be apart.

The baby may have some difficulty at first with digestion. If this is the case, try holding him over your shoulder and patting or rubbing his back, or lay him on his belly on your lap and stroke it. It can also help to massage his belly. In this case lay the baby on his back on your lap and gently but firmly press the abdomen with your fingers. Only continue if the baby seems to be enjoying it.

Babies love rhythm and body contact. Walking, rocking, swaying or gently bobbing up and down while holding the baby can help to soothe and comfort him. Babies love being sung and talked to or rocked to sleep. Baby slings or carriers which you can use to carry the child on your body are excellent and he will benefit from the warmth and the security of being close to you. You can begin to use these within a week or so of the birth. Babies also enjoy going for walks and if all else fails a drive in a car usually puts a baby to sleep.

It is impossible to 'spoil' a newborn baby by giving him too much love, contact or attention and letting a baby 'cry it out' is not a solution. Sometimes, however, a baby can be inconsolable for a while. In this case all one can do is to try one's best to comfort and satisfy the baby and hold him close to you until the crying passes.

Generally babies that are breastfed whenever they are hungry and have enough love and contact are contented and peaceful most of the time!

BATHING YOUR BABY

Having spent the months of pregnancy in the watery world of the womb, babies usually love to be in warm water. Bathing a baby is a very pleasant activity for the parents too. You can bath a baby any time from a few moments after birth. The purpose is more for relaxation and pleasure than for cleanliness. In some places where active birth is practised the baby is bathed in warm water by placing a bath between the mother's legs before the placenta is delivered in the third stage. This can be very relaxing and pleasurable for the baby, provided the bath is big enough and the water deep enough for him to float freely. Many parents love to take a baby with them into the water and bath together.

CHANGING YOUR BABY

The baby will urinate and empty his bowels often and a good supply of nappies and simple baby clothes is necessary. It is helpful to use disposable nappies in the early weeks. When changing a newborn baby it is a good idea to use a table on which everything you will need is placed within easy reach beforehand. Make sure that the room is warm. You will need a bowl of warm water and some cotton wool. Do not use synthetic creams, powders and lotions or baby products as these usually disturb the natural balance of oil and bacteria on the baby's skin. Simply wash the baby's genital area with warm water using cotton wool and then dry it very well, particularly in the creases, before putting on a fresh nappy. Give the baby time to stretch out and enjoy being changed and make use of this period to communicate and play with him.

Don't be surprised if a newborn baby hates being changed. This will pass as he becomes more familiar with an airy, unconfined environment. If this is the case it may help to place the baby in your lap while changing him and to keep him covered as much as possible. You needn't hesitate to use a firm but gentle touch. Although small babies look very delicate, in fact they are very strong and enjoy being handled fairly firmly. It will probably take you a few days before you feel completely relaxed and comfortable when handling your baby.

The first few bowel movements after birth are a dark green and black sticky substance called meconium which is in the baby's bowel in the womb. The colostrum and first milk help to clear this out of the baby's system and gradually over the first few days the colour lightens until it is the yellowish colour of a normal bowel movement.

Playful exercise

Babies love to be played with, handled, touched, talked, and sung to. A newborn baby, born without medication, is alert and responsive to the facial expressions of others and sensitive to the emotional states of those around him. In order to develop well and have a good start in life babies need plenty of love and physical contact.

Playful exercise provides the perfect opportunity for communication between an adult and a baby. It promotes the development of motor skills, balance, strength, flexibility and co-ordination, ensures good posture and self-confidence and also helps to dissipate stress.

Many parents are afraid to play with their babies in this way through fear of injuring them or ignorance of what a baby is capable of doing. By watching the process of development in your baby you can learn to handle him in a playful way which will stimulate his urge for movement and contact. You can discover a pleasurable physical dialogue with your baby which will encourage a relationship between you of co-operation, trust, ease, joy, and love.

Although the rate of development of a baby varies from child to child, there is a general pattern of growth which is universal. In the last few weeks in the womb the baby is curled up in a tight foetal position. After birth the baby transfers to an unconfined, airy environment and is subject to the force of gravity for the first time. To begin with the baby unfolds his body slowly. Then the development of muscular control starts from the top of the body downwards, beginning with the neck muscles. The newborn baby has very little control of his head. Gradually, as the neck muscles strengthen, the baby learns to hold his head up independently. After this the chest and upper back muscles strengthen and then the lower back and abdominal muscles develop co-ordination until finally the child can sit up with a straight back. The arms develop co-ordination before the legs and the baby can crawl, pulling himself forward with his arms, before he crawls properly on all-fours, which involves the use of his legs. After crawling the child will learn to squat, stand up and then finally, to walk.

The instructions that follow are an introduction to playful exercise between parent and child which can start from a few weeks after the birth and continue throughout childhood.

When to start

You can start just a few days after birth or whenever it feels right.

At first attempt only one or two movements, increasing gradually. The session should last no longer than four or five minutes to begin with, building up slowly to ten to fifteen minutes. Choose a time when your baby is alert, relaxed and ready for play. The best time is usually after a bath or during a nappy change but never just after feeding. Make sure you are comfortable and relaxed yourself and use a soft, gentle touch, which is firm but not sudden or jerky. Talk or sing to your baby while you play but always be ready to stop if he does not seem to be in the mood. Babies usually enjoy this sort of play enormously but it is important to allow them to lead the way and let their responses and pleasure be your guide.

Use slow, gentle movements and introduce each exercise gradually. Never attempt too much in one session. Your child should be without clothes in a warm room. You can support him in your hands, on your lap or else place him or her on a soft, clean surface while you play. Work on the floor if you can as your baby will enjoy having you at the same level. If your baby enjoys it, don't hesitate to stroke and massage his body gently at the same time.

How to handle your baby

First of all get to know the structure of your baby by gently stroking his body and feeling his muscles and bones.

Try different ways of holding your baby

* Sit crosslegged on the floor with your back supported and allow your baby to rest in your lap with his head on the inside of your knee and his body supported in the crook of your leg. In this position the baby is secure and you are free to use your arms and hands.
* If you do not like being on the floor, try sitting in a comfortable chair with the baby facing you on your lap, his head resting on your knees.
* A secure way of holding your baby is to use the palm and extended fingers of one hand to support the back of the head, while the palm and fingers of the other hand are spread around the baby's hips and along the spine.

EXERCISE 1

In this position observe the baby's head movements. See how he turns his head from side to side. Gradually you can encourage this movement by rotating the head to one side, bringing the baby's profile in line with the shoulder, your open hand spread comfortably under his head. Now wait until your child turns his head in the opposite direction before repeating the exercise.

EXERCISE 2

Also in this position, with one hand supporting the back of your baby's head and the other the hips and spine, press the chest gently forward with your fingers allowing the head, still supported, to go back. Then make the opposite movement, gently bringing the head forward towards the breastbone. Repeat a few times.

EXERCISE 3

Put the baby in your lap and gently turn the hips and legs first to the left and then to the right.

EXERCISE 4

Sit on the floor with your legs extended and together and your back supported. Alternatively, sit on a straight-backed chair. Place your baby on his back on your lap, his head resting on your knees. Bend your knees and allow your child's head to hang back gently over the edge, supporting his chest with one hand in front and the back of his head with your other hand. Lift the head up for a few seconds and then gently let it down, keeping your hand in position.

With your baby lying on his back, play with his hands and feet bending the joints back and forth at the wrists and ankles and allowing the baby to grip your fingers. Allow the baby to grip your thumb with his hands and open his arms out to the sides. Then slowly bring them together and cross them over the chest slowly and rhythmically. Repeat a few times.

After the baby learns to enjoy this movement, try bringing his arms up over and behind his head and down again to his side, first both arms together and then each in turn.

Hold up both feet with one hand at the ankles, placing your forefinger between the feet, so that the spine is gently raised off your lap while the head remains supported. Gently tickle first the lower, then the middle and upper back so that the baby arches and strengthens his spine.

EXERCISE 5

Place your baby on his belly on a soft, clean surface. Gently stroke his spine, making a slow and firm movement down from the neck to the lower back. In this position a newborn baby will lie with his head to one side, his pelvis raised and knees drawn up to the belly as if kneeling.

By one month the baby will lift his chin up momentarily and begin to kick, stretch and extend his legs. By two months the legs will be partly extended and straightened. Around three months the baby will be able to lift his chin and shoulders up for a long time, supporting its weight on the forearms with the legs fully extended.

Gently lift your baby up, supporting only the chest with your hands, one in front and one at the back. With a newborn baby the head will loll down. By about six weeks the baby will be able to lift his head up to be in line with his abdomen. This will increase by eight weeks until at three months the baby will be able to hold his head well up. This exercise strengthens the neck and shoulders.

EXERCISE 6   (Sit ups)

Lay your baby down on his back on a soft, clean surface. Hold the feet down gently with one hand, use your other hand to clasp both the baby's hands and gently bring him up to a sitting position. Hold for a few seconds and then gently lower the baby to the lying position.

EXERCISE 7   (Supported standing)

From four to eight weeks support your baby as if he were standing, with one hand supporting the upper back, neck and head and the other his chest. Allow the baby's weight to rest partially on the feet. The baby will probably make 'walking' or bouncing movements spontaneously but do not force this. Hold for a few seconds only and then rest. After ten weeks you can support your baby by gently holding both sides of the chest in your hands.

By the time your child is one year old he will have developed many motor skills. By the end of six months full head control will have been gained. At nine months the sitting position is completed as crawling and standing begin. At about eleven months a child can crawl, lean over, and twist while sitting. At the same time he will start to stand and walk with support.

Both the parents and the baby can have hours of pleasure together by continuing this playful exercise. At the same time you will be helping to ensure that your child has confidence, balance, strength, and flexibility which will form the foundations of health and physical wellbeing for the rest of his or her life. (For further reading on baby gymnastics see page 163.)

Further Reading

Balaskas, Arthur and Stirk, John, *Soft Exercise*, Unwin Paperbacks, 1983

Balaskas, Arthur and Walker, Peter, *Baby Gymnastics*, Unwin Paperbacks, not yet published

Balaskas, Janet, *Active Birth*, Unwin Paperbacks, 1983

Balaskas, Janet and Arthur, *New Life*, Sidgwick & Jackson, 1979 and 1983

Beels, Christine, *The Childbirth Book*, Turnstone Press, 1978

Brewer, G.S. and T., *What Every Woman Should Know: The Truth About Diet and Drugs in Pregnancy*, Random House, USA, 1977

Chard, Tim and Richards, Martin, *Benefits and Hazards of the New Obstetrics*, Heinemann Medical Books, 1977

Dick-Read, Grantly, *Childbirth Without Fear*, Pan Books, 1969

Flanagan, Geraldine Lux, *The First Nine Months of Life*, Heinemann Medical Books, 1963

Gaskin, Ina May, *Spiritual Midwifery*, The Book Publishing Co., USA, 1977

Haire, Doris, 'The Cultural Warping of Childbirth', *Environmental Child Health*, USA, vol.19, 171–91, June 1973

Kitzinger, Sheila, *Birth at Home*, Oxford University Press, 1979
Experience of Breast Feeding, Penguin Books, 1979
Experience of Childbirth, Penguin Books, 1970 and Gollancz, 1972
Giving Birth, Sphere, 1979
Good Birth Guide, Fontana, 1979
Women as Mothers, Fontana, 1978

Kitzinger, Sheila and Davis, John, *The Place of Birth*, Oxford University Press, 1978

La Leche League International, *The Womanly Art of Breastfeeding*, Souvenir Press, 1970 and Tandem, 1975

Leach, Penelope, *Baby and Child*, Michael Joseph, 1977 and Penguin Books, 1980

Leboyer, Frederick, *Birth Without Violence*, Fontana, 1977

Inner Beauty, Inner Light: Yoga for Pregnant Women, Alfred A. Knopf, USA, 1978

Loving Hands, Collins, 1977

Liedloff, Jean, *The Continuum Concept*, Duckworth, 1975 and Futura, 1976

Llewellyn-Jones, Derek, *Everywoman: A Gynaecological Guide for Life*, Faber and Faber, 1978

Montague, A., *Touching*, Columbia University Press, 1971

National Childbirth Trust, *Episiotomy – Physical and Emotional Aspects*, 1981

Nilsson, Lennart, *A Child is Born*, Faber and Faber, 1977

Stanway, Penny and Andrew, *Breast is Best*, Pan Books, 1978

Useful Addresses

The Active Birth Centre
  18 Laurier Road
  London
  NW5 1SG

Association for Improvement
in Maternity Services (AIMS)
  Christine Beels
  19 Broomfield Crescent
  Leeds 6
  and
  Elizabeth Cockerell
  10 Stonecliffe View
  Farnley
  Leeds LS12 5BE

Association of Radical
Midwives (ARM)
  Lakefield
  8a The Drive
  Wimbledon
  London SW20 8TG

The Birth Centre
  16 Simpson Street
  London SW11 3HN

British Homoeopathic
Association
  Basildon Court
  27a Devonshire Street
  London W1N 1RT

La Leche League, Great Britain
(Breastfeeding counsellors)
  Box 3424
  London WC1 6XX

The Meet-a-Mum Association
(MAMA)
  Mary Whitlock
  26a Cumnor Hill
  Oxford OX2 9HA

National Childbirth Trust
  9 Queensborough Terrace
  London W2 3TB

National Council for One-
Parent Families
  255 Kentish Town Road
  London NW5 2LX

The Patients Association
  Room 33
  18 Charing Cross Road
  London WC2H 0HR

Society to Support Home
Confinements
  Margaret Whyte
  17 Laburnam Avenue
  Durham

For classes in the Balaskas method of preparation for
Active Birth, contact:

The Active Birth Movement
  18 Laurier Road
  London
  NW5 1SG
  01-267-3006

Index